DR. SEBI DIET:

A 7-Days Diet to Lose Weight, Cleanse Liver, Reduce Risk of Diseases, Detox Your Body, and Become Healthier with Alkaline Food Recipes and Herbs

Table of Contents

Introduction

Congratulations on taking the first steps to improve your health by choosing the Dr. Sebi Treatment and Cures Book. In this book, you will learn all of the healing secrets of Dr. Sebi and how they can help you to improve your health.

This is why in this book, we are going to take a closer look at some cogent points made by Dr. Sebi. The Honduran herbalist, Dr. Sebi is well revered for positively changing the lives of many around the world with his herbal knowledge. These so-called changes were made possible by an alkaline diet which he tagged "African Bio-Electric Cell Food Therapy."

Choosing alkaline foods is the only way to live and lose extra pounds for healthy living.

It's believed to rebuild your cells through removing radioactive waste by alkalizing the blood. Dr. Sebi was not a surgeon, considering his position, and did not possess a PhD.

He developed this diet for those seeking to treat or avoid diseases and enhance their general wellbeing without focusing on traditional Western medication.

Dr. Sebi's diet is not approved by official sources and no scientific evidence shows that medical conditions can be prevented or treated using this method.

Chapter 1: Who is Dr. Sebi?

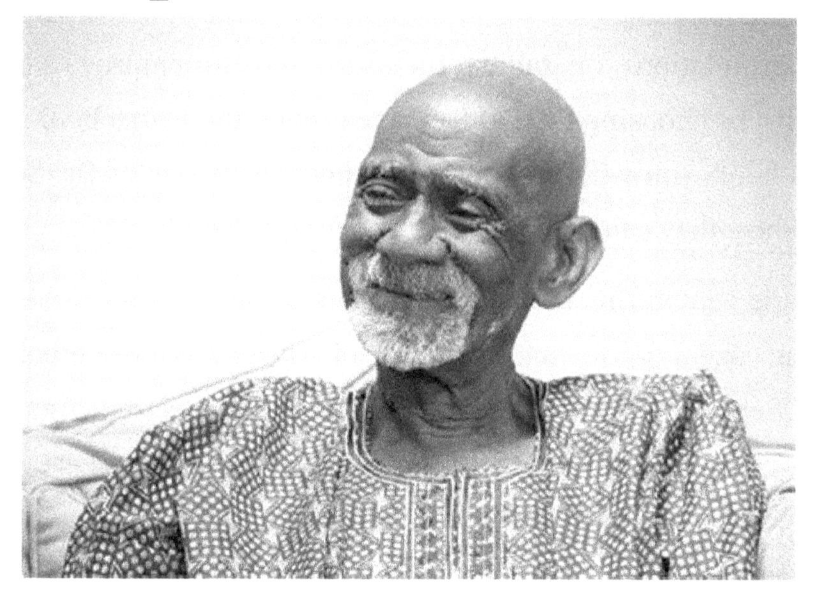

The man behind the Dr. Sebi Diet is Alfredo Bowman. He is a Honduran self-proclaimed herbalist and healer who uses food to improve health. Although he is already deceased, he has a number of followers in the 21st century. Because of his holistic approach, he has claimed to cure many kinds of diseases using herbs and a strict vegan diet. He has set up a treatment center in his home country before moving to New York City, where he has continued his practice and extended his clienteles to Michael Jackson, John Travolta, Eddie Murphy, and Steven Seagal, to name a few.

Although he calls himself Dr. Sebi, he does not hold any medical nor Ph.D. degree. Moreover, the diet has claimed to cure different conditions such as sickle-cell anemia, lupus, leukemia, and HIV-AIDS. This led to a lot of issues, particularly that he was practicing medicine without a license and his exorbitant claims. While he was charged for practicing without a license, he was acquitted in the early 1990s due to a lack of evidence. However, he was instructed to stop making claims that his diet can treat HIV-AIDS. While there are controversies that surround his name, there are so many benefits of his alkaline vegan diet that it are still popular even to this date.

The Dr. Sebi Alkaline Eating Diet

Dr. Sebi believed that acidity and mucus could cause different types of diseases. For instance, the buildup of mucus in the lungs can lead to pneumonia. He noted that eating certain types of food, and avoiding others like the plague, can help detoxify the body. It can also bring the body to an alkaline state that can reduce the risk of developing many types of diseases. By turning the blood alkaline, the cells can be rejuvenated and can easily eliminate toxins out. Moreover, he argues that diseases cannot exist in an environment that is alkaline. His principle of making the body more alkaline is what other plant-based diets are banking on.

This particular diet relies on eating a list of approved foods as well as the intake of certain types of supplements. For the body to heal itself, Dr. Sebi noted that this diet should be followed consistently for the rest of your life.

The Dr. Sebi Diet is plant-based, but unlike other plant-based diets, there are some differences in this diet compared to the plant-based diet in general. Here is a compiled list of what differentiates the Dr. Sebi Diet from a plant-based diet.

No processed foods

Tofu, veggie burgers, textured vegetable protein, canned fruits, canned vegetables, oil, soy sauce, and other condiments are considered processed. The Dr. Sebi Diet encourages dieters to consume food that is unadulterated. Some plant-based diets still allow the consumption of processed foods, as long as they are made from plant-based ingredients.

No wheat products allowed

Under this diet regimen, you are not allowed to consume wheat and wheat products such as bread, biscuits, and others as they are not naturally-grown grains. Naturally-grown grains include amaranth seeds, wild rice, and triticale, to name a few.

The need to adhere to the food list

In general, plant-based diets are not so restrictive when it comes to the food that dieters are allowed to eat (unless you are specifically following a strict plant-based regimen such as the plant-based keto diet). However, the Dr. Sebi Diet requires dieters to only eat foods that are listed in the nutritional guide.

Drink one (1) gallon of water daily

Water is the most hydrating liquid on the planet. The Dr. Sebi Diet requires dieters to consume 1 gallon of water daily or more. Moreover, tea and coffee should be avoided as these drinks are highly acidic.

Taking Dr. Sebi's supplements

If you are taking any medications for a particular health condition, this particular diet regimen will require you to consume proprietary supplements an hour before taking your medication.

What Was the Diet Based On?

He believed that the diseases inside our body are caused by the buildup of mucus in different organs—like if the heart had a buildup of mucus, it leads to heart disease, and if it is in excess in the pancreas, it causes diabetes. He also claimed that diseases thrive in acidic environments and die in an alkaline environment. He said that the diet would restore the body's original healthy start if we strictly follow it and consume the mixtures/supplements that he originally made. The body will then be cleansed and detoxified of harmful substances. Natural foods mentioned in this diet are high in alkalinity, and it raises the body pH, so according to Alfredo's theories, they can heal the body by creating an alkaline environment internally.

The diet is made up of lists of different vegetables, fruits, seeds, grains, nuts, and oils, with no addition of animal-sourced food. That is why the diet can also be considered a vegan diet. However, it is even more restrictive than that as some vegetables, grains, and fruits are banned from being consumed. For example, you are not permitted to eat seedless fruits in this diet. Also, to get the maximum and continuous benefit, Dr. Sebi says to follow this diet for the entirety of your life, which makes the diet even more strict and restrictive.

Dr. Sebi's Teachings and Methods

Dr. Sebi proposed that the body is at the state of becoming susceptible to contracting diseases when the level of toxins and mucus accumulation increases. He argued that people that are suffering from different diseases and those that are interested in preventing diseases should always eat an alkaline diet, bearing in mind that when the body removes the increased amount of acidic substances and mucus, it becomes free from infections.

He also suggested that cleansing and detoxification of the body is an essential and significant tool necessary in dealing with any form of the disease in the body.

Detoxification of the body assists in the elimination of mucus accumulated in the liver, lungs, and many other body organs and also helps in the removal of excess acidic substances, thereby making the body free from disease-causing diseases.

Dr. Sebi also made use of herbs that are important in re-energizing and revitalizing the body. The organs of the body function properly when there is an improvement in your health, and this indicates that your body is void of diseases.

Some Disadvantages of Doctor Sebi Diet You Must Know

The alkaline diet by Dr. Sebi has a lot of disadvantages too.

The following is a list of the disadvantages:

Highly restrictive:

The diet's main con is that it hinders businesses that specialize in foods such as wheat, animal products, lentils, beans, and many other varieties of fruits and vegetables.

The diet only allows specific fruit forms. An example is consuming plum or cherry tomatoes but not other forms like thc Roma or beefsteak tomatoes.

As the diet harshly criticizes ingredients that are not found in nutrition manuals, one can develop a negative attitude towards food. You will realize that following the diet is not always fun.

Lastly, the weight-loss plan can encourage some bad behaviors and the use of supplements. The supplements are usually not the best source of calories. As a result, one ends up having poor styles of consuming foods.

Absence of proteins and other important vitamins:

Listed ingredients in the diet plan of Dr. Sebi can also act as good sources of vitamins.

Nonetheless, not the certified foods can be the source of proteins, important nutrients for skin and pore structure, hormone, and enzymes production, and muscle boom.

The only certified foods that have the proteins mentioned are hemp seeds, walnuts, Brazil nuts, and sesame seeds.

To obtain the daily required proteins, you need to consume large amounts of the doctor's ingredients.

The ingredients have a high concentration of nutrients like: potassium, nutrient C and E, beta, and carotene. They have a low concentration of ingredients like iron, omega-3, vitamins B12 and D, and calcium.

Dr. Sebi Classification of Food

Dr. Sebi classified food into six categories.

These categories are:

- Drugs.

- Genetically modified foods.
- Hybrid foods.
- Dead foods.
- Living foods.
- Raw foods.

He concluded that the first four categories of food in this list are no-go areas as they cause more damage in the body than good. These foods can cause a buildup of acids and mucus in the body. However, the last two categories of foods are the best types of food he classified as healthy because the nutritional contents in them are not lost in any way. For instance, foods that are thoroughly cooked, hybridized, and modified have lost the required amount of nutrients present in them. Hence, instead of providing benefits for the body, the reverse is the case. However, raw foods, especially vegetables, fruits, and herbs, are excellent for building good health.

Information about Dr. Sebi's Diet

Dr. Sebi's diets are diets that are plant-based and electric in nature. Dr. Sebi's diets are African biomineral diets which help dieters to fight diseases. The diet also serves as the prevention of various diseases (prophylaxis) and helps in boosting the immune system. When the body is immuno-compromised, it is said to accommodate any infection that sneaks in.

Dr. Sebi's diet is also beneficial for people who cherish to live a healthy life by remaining clean and lean. His diet was not created from Heaven; they are common foods we ignore because of the love of modified, processed, refined, and hybridized foods.

Dr. Sebi's diet contains vegetables, fruits, grains, nuts, herbal teas, plant-based sweeteners, and seeds. Those who cherish animal products will not benefit from this diet as it does not encourage foods that are made from animals.

According to Dr. Sebi, all infections grow well in the environment that makes them comfortable such as acidic, mucus overload, and toxic environs.

When the body is in a limy condition, infections will find it so difficult to thrive, and when it is in an acidic state, the reverse is the case. Hence, the acidic component in the body helps diseases to multiply and thrive.

Likewise, he also declared that the buildup of excess mucus in the body increases the susceptibility of having an infection as the mucus block up the blood vessel and hinders the flow of blood easily.

He stated that the excess mucus must be removed for you to enjoy your health. When the mucus is removed either by detoxification or cleansing, the diseases are automatically removed.

The diets of Dr. Sebi have been proven effective by those who truly love them. The diets re-energize and revitalize the body by bringing it back to its normal state.

The healing of many sufferers who suffers from hair loss and many other prevalent diseases didn't occur because of the medications they took but because of the self-healing that took place in the body due to the intake of Dr. Sebi's alkaline diet.

The benefits of the diet will be explained later on, but it should be clear that it is a restrictive diet, low in calories. Many people believe that because of this reason, it cannot be used as a standard way to lose weight as it puts too much stress on the body of a new dieter. Because it is low in calories and is an intensive diet, weight loss can be seen, but the person needs to assess whether they are capable of handling a low caloric diet. Being too ambitious with this diet might turn fatal, so if you want to try the diet, be careful!

This diet has been suggested to be followed throughout one's entire life, which might not be possible for a new dieter. With any diet, if you start cutting foods strongly and then revert to your old routine of eating unhealthy meals, the chances are that the weight loss and benefits you see will get reversed. This is a risk in this diet as well. When starting, set reasonable goals and don't go too strongly. Let your body first get used to it and then start setting up more ambitious goals.

Who is the Alkaline Diet For?

Due to the move in the populace to a diet higher in acid, individuals who have specific indications should attempt the alkaline diet to check whether it makes a difference. These manifestations include:

- Individuals who have no energy
- At the point when the body delivers an excess of bodily fluid
- Clogged nose
- Individuals who have incessant influenza and colds
- Individuals who are on edge, apprehensive and bad-tempered
- Individuals who have ovarian growths, polycystic ovaries, and amiable bosom sores
- Individuals who have incessant cerebral pains or headaches

Benefits of Dr. Sebi Treatments

Dr. Sebi's Diet offers a lot of benefits to the dieters. While the foods recommended from this diet are known to reduce inflammation, there are other benefits that you can reap from following the Dr. Sebi Diet.

May Help with Weight Loss

While this diet regimen is not designed for weight loss, it can help people who want to lose weight. Studies show that people who consume an unlimited whole plant-based diet experience significant weight loss company. How people lose weight with this diet relies on the high fiber and low-calorie foods that you are encouraged to eat. Except for avocadoes, nuts, seeds, and oil, most foods encouraged by the Dr. Sebi Diet are low in calories. But even if you consume nuts and seeds, they are not only calorie-dense but also rich in fiber and minerals.

Better Colon Health

Because this diet regimen encourages the consumption of large volumes of fruits and vegetables, it also has benefits to colon health. Foods rich in fiber can help promote healthy digestion; thus, people who follow the Dr. Sebi Diet do not suffer from constipation.

Appetite Control

Although many people think that this diet is very restrictive in terms of the number of calories a particular person takes in, studies are indicating that this diet can help with appetite control. The high fiber in your food can provide a high satiety level and can make one feel full for much longer.

Improves kidney function

Acidic diets mostly affect the health of the kidneys and damages the layers inside the organ system. To promote kidney health, the pH of the urine mustn't be acidic. By consuming a lot of alkaline food and removing acidic foods from our daily routine, we can reach this pH in which our kidneys remain safe and healthy. Alkaline diets do not affect the pH of the blood, but it can significantly affect the urine. Drinking a lot of water alongside this diet can improve kidneys even more.

Reduces the risk of cancer

There are almost no significant studies that show that an alkaline diet leads to decreased cases of cancer. However, there have been studies that show that if a person were to eat less meat and increase their consumption of fresh fruits and vegetables, then that person is at a lower risk of cancer.

Reduces the risk of heart disease

Heart disease is a major cause of death in the world. It is mainly caused by eating lots of fat and oily foods, which results in the development of plaque and blockage of arteries. In this diet, the consumption of fats goes down significantly, decreasing the chances of developing heart disease.

Solid Immune System

A powerless and vulnerable framework is the consequence of ailments and diseases. Some cases that they have fortified their insusceptible framework and have been mended of specific sicknesses by following the Dr. Sebi diet reliably. We, as a whole, realize that medication doesn't fix diseases.

Diminished Risk of Disease

Acidic nourishments dissolve the mucus film of the cells and internal dividers of the body, which prompts an undermined framework that makes disease conceivable and a fix inconceivable. Accordingly, eating alkaline nourishments can diminish the danger of illness and help your body in getting what it needs to encourage high cells.

Lower Risk of Stroke and Hypertension

As indicated by the National Institute of Health (NIH), first-line treatments for all phases of hypertension incorporate exercise and weight loss. In any case, results from one microscopic cross-sectional examination propose that a plant-based diet is a more significant intercession than medication and standard therapeutic practice. Regular Health has additionally talked about the advantages of a plant-based diet in contrast with medicine, expressing that a plant-based diet can diminish plaque in the veins and lower the danger of diabetes, stroke, and coronary illness in restorative research they have investigated.

Energy

Diets overwhelming in meat, dairy, and white sugar can be a drag on your body and energy levels. Concentrating on plant-based living is a superior approach and can upgrade the energy that you show all the time.

Expanded Focus

Following Dr. Sebi's lessons will clear the cerebrum haze, keeping you engaged and less annoyed by upsetting circumstances that emerge. Regardless of whether you are not wiped out, utilizing a plant-based methodology will assist you with carrying on with a long and healthy life.

Reduces the risk of muscle degradation

When we grow old or stop using our muscles, we tend to increase muscle loss. However, there was a study conducted in 2013 showing that people who follow the alkaline diet could decrease muscle degradation. The diet is low in red meat, so there is a risk of decreasing muscle mass and strength.

People eat more fruits and vegetables

Nowadays, people lean towards the fast and tasty treats and forget about eating fresh produce. Following this diet will lead to people consuming their daily requirement of vegetables and fruits. With the increase in their intake, we take in all their benefits and nutrition as well.

Increases intestinal health

With the addition of whole grains, there is a list of nuts and seeds that you can eat on this diet. It contributes to an increase in fiber intake, which increases the health of small and large intestines. It helps manage regular bowel movements, which reduces the risk of developing many diseases.

Decreases the harmful effects of processed foods

Processed foods have been linked to increased sugar intake and fat content. They also contain lots of calories but have very low nutritional value. Many additives and preservatives that have no purpose in our body are eliminated from our diets if we strictly avoid processed foods.

It helps the brain

The growth hormone is not only related to a better heart condition but also helps manage the health of the mind. It is related to an increase in memory and cognition. Eating a healthy diet rich in fruits and vegetables leads to better brain functioning.

It may improve back pain

Alkaline minerals are related to the reduction of back pain, but whether alkaline foods provide the same results has yet to be determined. There is a decent chance that the diet has similar effects.

Decreases the level of inflammation

Diets rich in fresh fruits and vegetables show a great decrease in oxidative stress and inflammation. This leads to less discomfort and fewer diseases developing in our bodies.

Better gut microbiome

The stomach is the second brain. The enzymes and molecules released by the microbes in the gut affect not only your health but even your everyday mood. What you put inside your system also affects the kinds of molecules that the microbes release into the bloodstream. The type of food that you also consume can also affect the kind of microbes in your stomach. For instance, studies show that consumption of greasy, fatty, and processed foods can lead to the decline of good microorganisms and promote the growth of bad bacteria in the body.

Reduced Inflammation

While inflammation is one of the body's first lines of defense indicating the presence of infection and diseases, chronic low-dose inflammation can also be bad to the body. In fact, the presence of chronic inflammation can result in many kinds of diseases such as diabetes, stroke, and even cancer. Thus, diets that are rich in fruits and vegetables are linked to reduced inflammation caused by oxidative stress.

Rules of Dr. Sebi

As you may have noticed, the Dr. Sebi diet is not like any other. Where other diets either have a bunch of information that you can't figure out what it means, Dr. Sebi's diet is very straightforward. You have the food list that you have to stick with, you have the supplements that you should take, and then you have the rules we are going to go over. While the diet does require giving up a lot of stuff, it is very easy to see what you should and should not do, which, in the long run, makes it easier to follow. Let's take a look at the rules.

You are only allowed to eat the foods that are listed on the nutritional guide.

The nutritional guide is the only guide you have for this diet, and those foods are the only approved foods. It really can't get any more straightforward than that. The only things that aren't really listed on the nutritional guide that you do get to consume are herbs that are most often used in supplements. Any herb that is used in Dr. Sebi's supplements, you can use in other ways as well, such as sea moss, burdock, and bladderwrack. You won't find those things on the nutritional guide, but they can be consumed in various ways and not just through the supplements.

You have to consume a gallon of water each day.

That may sound like a lot, but with some planning, you can do it. Just so you know, a gallon of water comes out to 3.8 liters. Your body is made up of mostly water and it needs water to work properly. There are so many people walking around who are dehydrated and dehydration has the power to make you feel awful. Dehydration can cause you to faint, feel fatigued or irritable, look tired, breathe quickly, have a rapid heartbeat, feel dizzy, have dry skin, and so much more. While some of these only happen in severe cases of dehydration, like fainting, the other symptoms are so common that people don't even think anything about it.

You are not allowed to consume any type of animal products.

The Dr. Sebi diet is very much a vegan alkaline diet. Our body does not have to have animal products to function. First off, we are the only mammals who feed their young milk from other mammals. Cows do not ask a goat for their milk to feed their babies. Then there is the act of eating meat. If you look at any carnivorous animals out there, such as lions, bears, or wolves, they all have sharp pointy canines and claws. Humans have small canine teeth and soft fingernails. Carnivores are provided the tools they need in order to tear flesh without the need for forks and knives. Their jaws also only move up and down, which gives them the ability to tear chunks of meat out of the prey. Humans can also move their jaw from side to side and we have flat molars, which are something carnivores do not have, and they allow us to grind up veggies and fruit just like herbivores.

You cannot consume alcohol.

Alcohol, as we all know, is very detrimental to our health, especially our liver. Alcohol is also very acidic. The liver has the hard job of breaking down harmful chemicals, and alcohol is only made up of harmful chemicals. When the liver has to work overtime in getting rid of alcohol, it can lead to cirrhosis, jaundice, and hepatitis. Alcohol is a waste product that the body wants to get, and the smallest amount affects the body. If you consume more alcohol than the body can process, you start to become intoxicated as it builds up. This will slow down how your body functions, including the immune system. This is why heavy drinkers are more likely to develop illnesses and it also increases their risk of several different types of cancer.

Do not use the microwave to cook your food because it will kill it.

Microwave ovens were made for convenience, and convenient they are, but they aren't really good for you or your food. Microwaves turn electricity into electromagnetic waves, which are called microwaves. This makes the molecules in your food vibrate and spin, which is what makes them hot. If you rub your hands together really fast, you will be doing, basically, the same thing. The microwave does produce a type of radiation, but there are a lot of protective factors on the microwave itself that keeps the radiation from reaching you, as long as the microwave is still in good condition.

You cannot consume seedless or canned fruits.

If you look up a definition of fruit, you would get something like "the sweet and fleshy product of a tree or other plant that contains seeds and can be eaten as food." By that definition, for a food to be considered a fruit, it has to contain seeds. That means seedless fruits aren't even fruits. Why is it normal to eat fruits that don't contain seeds? You've likely had both the seeded and seedless varieties of foods and probably can't even notice a difference. But seedless fruits are not okay. They aren't even able to reproduce. The process that fruits go through to make them seedless creates something that our bodies don't even recognize, so they aren't able to use them.

You should not consume foods that are hybrid.

Hybrid and crossbreeding foods is the act of making a new plant by combining two or more species. The new species will have characteristics of their parents but is also their own unique food. This was started as a way to create plants that could be controlled or cultivated. The new species is able to live in places and conditions that its parents couldn't. This is how our modern wheat was created. By changing up the genetic order of a plant, it causes the starch content to increase, which tends to be very corrosive to human tissue.

Changing the genetic order of foods causes chemical and genetic mineral imbalances.

Hybrid foods will not grow in nature. They are simply a product of man and have to be constantly protected and nurtured by humans. Hybrid foods have been removed from their natural content and cannot assimilate in the body and will only cause you to store toxins.

You cannot consume coffee or sodas, only spring water and herbal teas.

Coffee, while not innately bad for your body, is also not all that great for you either. The caffeine in coffee is addictive, which causes people to crave more caffeine. The more you drink, the higher your tolerance for it grows and the more you need to get the high you are looking for. Somebody also finds that coffee hurts their stomach and digestive tract, and can also lead to heartburn and stomach ulcers. While it can be hard to give up coffee, it will be worth it in the long run because you will be allowing your natural energy to return without the need for caffeine.

What Is the Result of the Diet?

The human body has a range of pH in which it gives optimum performance. It is slightly alkaline, with a range of 7.25–7.35. Many alkaline diets like this one promise to help the body maintain these slightly alkaline levels. In reality, it does almost nothing to the pH levels of the blood because the body has a built-in process to keep it under control. Regardless, following an alkaline diet leads to many health benefits as it encourages the consumption of fruits and vegetables, unprocessed fresh products, and discourages the use of alcohol and other potentially harmful substances. It also makes you drink lots of water.

This diet results in steady weight loss, decreases the risks of many diseases, and lowers the chances of developing them. Kidney stones and kidney diseases are less frequent. Bones and muscles get stronger. It results in higher functioning of the heart and brain, also lowering the chances of their deterioration. You are less likely to develop type 2 diabetes as it is related to obesity, and this diet helps remove obesity by effective weight loss.

People who believe in Dr. Sebi's diet say that it reduces the built-up acidity in our bodies. If we stop eating alkaline foods, the acid will start to accumulate, and our body will attract many types of diseases. Eating a constant influx of alkaline foods helps to reduce diseases and acidity.

Who Could Benefit from this Diet?

Almost anyone looking to better their life can follow this diet. Unhealthy eating has become prominent all over the world. People of all ages prefer to practically run away from vegetables and fruits these days. Apart from some popular ingredients, people don't know about the large variety of foods that are available at their disposal. Because of laziness and ignorance, people choose not to look at all of the options that might greatly benefit them and settle for the easiest thing they can get on the plate. Dieting, especially alkaline dieting, which is mainly focused on vegetables and fruits, is a crucial step in improving people's health.

More people are obese than ever before. Heart disease and diabetes are the major causes of death. All these aspects are related to bad eating and can be improved if we switch to a healthy and nutritious eating routine, just like this diet.

The people that can benefit the most are obese people looking for a way to shed some pounds so that they don't invite diseases into their bodies. The diet effectively makes a person lose weight and reach their weight goals, so obese and overweight people can improve their lives significantly. Also, it can help people suffering from heart disease and diabetes. Still, before patients should opt for the diet, it is advised that they seek the guidance of a health professional before adopting such a restrictive and low caloric diet.

Reviews About the Diet

Many people have tried and commented on their diet. The people who started the diet were mostly people looking for an effective weight-loss method. The dieting plan ranges from about four weeks for some people with probably a cheat day or two. A complete strict adaptation of the diet for your whole life, just as you are starting, is a near-impossible thing to do even if you have high motivation.

People switching to the diet for the first time—whose meals consist of meat, rice, and bread, with occasional snacking—found the diet to be very difficult during the first week. Their daily routine was affected as they felt a loss in energy, and they sensed weakness for the first few days. Dieters who took supplements and planned their meals to be rich in calories found that they gained some of their energy back, but it was still not enough. After weeks three and four, the diet became easier to follow. In the end, dieters on average saw a great reduction in their weight—approximately two to four pounds per day, after five or six weeks of dieting was completed.

For most people, shopping for the ingredients was quite expensive. You have to buy whole grain, vegetables, fruits, and also supplements that don't make it financially sustainable. It is already a restrictive diet, which makes the dieter lose motivation even further.

There was a concern about malnutrition among dieters. Because this diet cuts off all sources of protein and other compounds like Vitamin B12, they had to take additional supplements.

Chapter 2: The Importance of Alkaline Water and Fruits

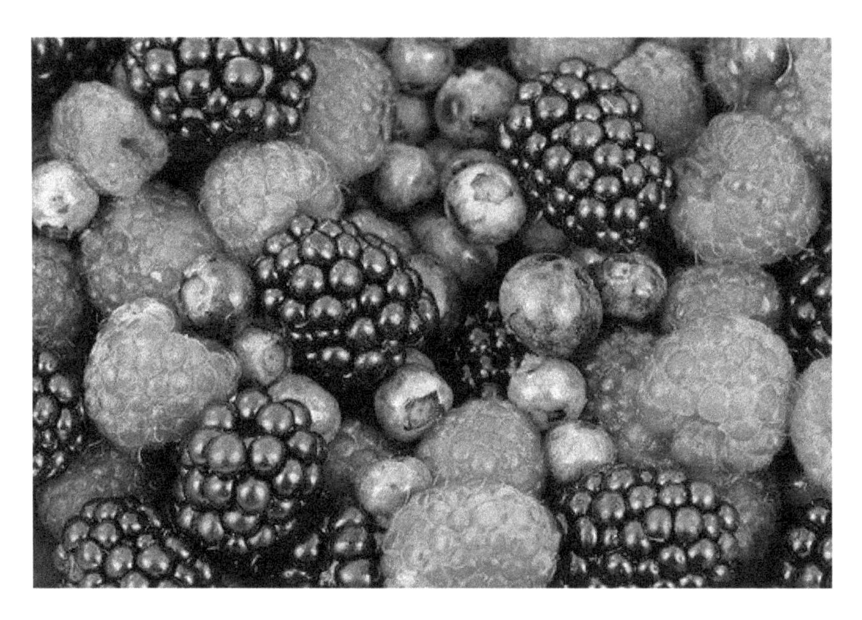

Give protection to bone density and muscle mass

Taking minerals into your body system plays a significant role in maintaining and developing the bones in your body. Research has proved to the truth that the more alkaline-rich fruits and vegetables you take regularly, the better you get protected from experiencing reduced bone muscle and strength known as Sarcopenia. What an alkaline diet does when you take it is to help in balancing the ratios of the various minerals in the body necessary for the bone-building and the maintenance of a lean muscle mass. The minerals that an alkaline diet balances are Phosphate, Magnesium, and Calcium. Another benefit of an alkaline diet in this regard is the improvement in the production of vitamin D absorption and growth hormones which helps in further protecting the bones and fighting against many chronic diseases.

Reduce the risk of hypertension and stroke

Another great benefit of eating an alkaline diet is the reduction of the risk of stroke and hypertension and individual is prone to have. A typical alkaline diet has an anti-aging effect. A robust result of the anti-aging effects is that it drastically reduces inflammation and fosters the growth of hormone production. This has been verified to help in the improvement of cardiovascular health and giving the body defense against typical health challenges like hypertension, high cholesterol, stroke, kidney stones, and possible memory loss.

Reduce chronic pain and inflammation

There is a correlation between alkaline diets and a drastic reduction in levels of chronic pain. Chronic acidosis is dangerous to the human health system. It is the primary cause of headaches, chronic back pain, joint pain, inflammation, menstrual symptoms, and muscle spasms.

Cases abound that show the health benefits of alkaline diets suffering from chronic pains. A study conducted showed that there was a significant level of decrease in the pain experienced by patients suffering from chronic back pain when they were supplements containing alkaline daily for four weeks.

Prevent deficiency in magnesium and increases vitamin absorption

Magnesium plays an essential role in the human body as an increase in its quantity is necessary for the proper functioning of all the enzymes and processes in the human body. Deficiency in magnesium content will result in headaches, anxiety, heart complications, muscle pains, and sleep troubles. Magnesium is also needed by the body in the activation of vitamin D and preventing Vitamin D deficiency, necessary for the functioning of the endocrine and overall body immunity.

Improving cancer protection and immune function

Minerals are needed by the body in disposing of waste or in oxygenating the body. But when there is a shortage of the required minerals in the cells, the body suffers. Vitamin absorption is zeroed off whenever there is a mineral loss in the body. Also, toxins and pathogens will pile up in the body thereby weakening the immune system. But with alkaline diets, that cannot happen as research has proved that the death of cancerous cells happens more in an alkaline body. Alkaline diets will help in decreasing inflammation and the possible risks associated with dangerous diseases such as cancer.

Help you in maintaining a healthy balanced weight

When you eat more of alkaline diets, you are not just limiting the acidic content in your body but also protecting your body from the risks associated with obesity. This is possible as alkaline diets decrease the levels of Leptin and inflammation which has a direct effect on your hunger and fat-burning capacities. Just like I have established to you that alkaline foods are anti-inflammatory foods, eating alkaline diets will give your body the possibility of attaining the ideal Leptin levels and prevent you from consuming too many calories.

Best Alkaline Foods Powerful for Boosting Your Health

Alkaline water

The PH level of alkaline water is always at a rate of 9 to 11. Distilled water is the ideal water for your body system in maintaining weight, health, and vitality. Water that has undergone the process of purification through reverse osmosis is a little acidic, though better than tap water. But alkaline water is the best in promoting alkalinity in the bloodstream. You can easily boost the alkalinity of your water by adding the following substances to it: (i) Lime (ii) Lemon (iii) Baking soda (iv) pH drops

Plant Proteins

Typical plant proteins include lima beans, almonds, and navy beans. The other common beans are also good as they help in promoting alkalinity in the bloodstream.

Green drinks

Green drinks refer to drinks that have been made from the combination of grasses and green vegetables in powdery form loaded with alkaline-rich foods and chlorophyll. Chlorophyll helps in alkalinizing the blood.

All raw foods

Raw fruits and vegetables are very healthy. They are biogenic, thereby life-giving. Cooked foods reduce the alkalinizing minerals in the body. It is therefore recommended that you improve on your intake of raw foods as they boost alkalinity. You can also juice or stream your vegetables and fruits.

Fresh fruits and vegetables

Fresh fruits and vegetables help in promoting the alkalinity level in your bloodstream and body. They have been proven to be the best in boosting alkalinity. Dr. Sebi recommended fresh fruits and vegetables to eat include the following: (i) Dates (ii) Mushrooms (iii) Citrus (iv) Avocado (v) Tomatoes (vi) Grapefruit (vii) Spinach (viii) Alfalfa grass (ix) Kale (x) Cucumber (xi) Ginger (xii) Garlic (xiii) Cabbage (xiv) Endive (xv) Green beans (xvi) Watermelon (xvii) Beets (xviii) Ripe bananas (xix) Figs (xx) Jicama (xxi) Celery (xxii) Oregano (xxiii) Broccoli (xxiv) Spinach (xxv) Summer black radish 6. Other best alkaline foods you should try to include: (i) Kamut (ii) Wheatgrass (iii) Sprouts (iv) Fermented Soy

Chapter 3: Dr. Sebi's Approach to Disease

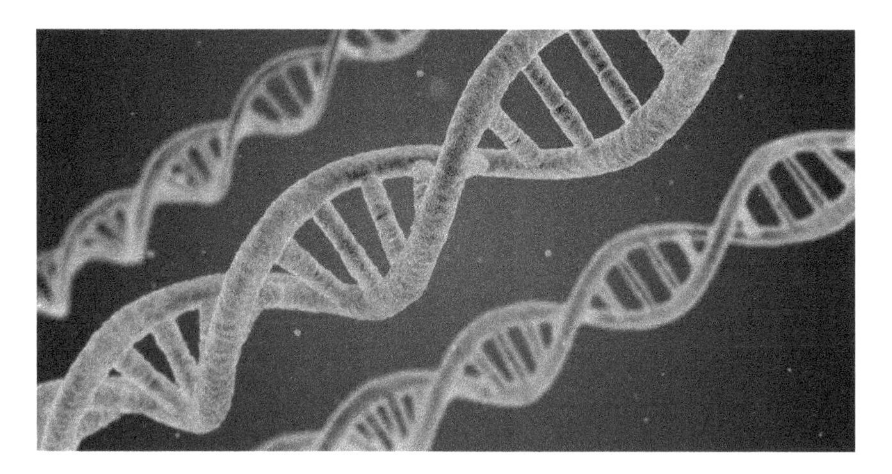

Diet and Disease

There is some proof that such a diet is useful in anticipating osteoporosis and other bone health issues. In any case, the evidence isn't substantial in supporting the instances that an alkaline diet may forestall or help lighten conditions, for example, cancer, weakness, heftiness, or sensitivities. There is, in any case, some proof that cancer cells develop all the more rapidly in an acidic situation in a research center setting. In this manner, an individual with an inclination to or who experiences this disease might need to research the impacts an alkaline diet has on the body.

Considering the mind-boggling ascend in a large number of these sorts of diseases, it is anything but difficult to think about whether they are brought about by the general state of an individual's interior body condition. A more extensive and all the more deductively fiery assessment of the Alkaline Diet is altogether. Be that as it may, such logical examination might be polluted from the earliest starting point by partiality instigated in a pharmaceutical-based health care delivery framework.

The theory behind the Alkaline Diet isn't broadly acknowledged by the therapeutic network, which might be one reason cancer, diabetes, and any number of other awful diseases are at pandemic levels. The Alkaline Diet, when joined with a physically dynamic, low-pressure way of life, surely merits more consideration from established researchers if they can keep their predisposition under control.

It would be generally easy to check whether specific conditions, for example, glucose, pulse, cholesterol tally, and an individual's weight standardize when (and if) their blood pH falls into the ideal range. These indications happen together so regularly that the medicinal network has started calling it Syndrome X. If this syndrome is so healthy and the convention for logical assessment so necessary, for what reason is the Alkaline Diet still, for example, riddle about whether it is valuable or not?

It might be because there is no cash to be produced using prescribing a particular diet. Pharmaceutical organizations test new drugs because there is a benefit to be made if the drug makes it advertise. Be that as it may, there is no benefit in dietary suggestions. In this way, such research would tumble to the colleges and administrative organizations to direct. The idea that the more significant part of those analysts likewise fills in as experts for the pharmaceutical business may effectively spoil their eagerness and discoveries.

Dr. Sebi: Natural Erectile Dysfunctions Cure

To cure the root cause of erectile dysfunction according to Dr. Sebi, there are 2 steps that cannot be avoided if you desire results. However, these steps are

Cleansing

Cleansing has to do with getting rid of mucus or detoxifying the body system using spring water, alkaline fruits smoothies, Irish sea moss, and the cleansing herbs.

Revitalizing

Revitalizing has to do with nourishing and replenishing of the body system and strengthening the immune system from the energy or damage that it has suffered as a result of the disease that it has suffered from.

Dieting

Although the steps are just the first two steps, Dr. Sebi stated that a lot of people were not able to be free from disease completely because after the cleansing and revitalizing process, they now return to eating acidic food that is making them vulnerable to disease again. However, dieting is changing your eating habit. That is, eating foods from Dr. Sebi's nutritional guide (I will talk about that soon).

Dr. Sebi Principles of Diabetes Nutrition

A majority of diabetic patients do not know the level of the nutrition taken advantage or forms side effects for them. Therefore, it is important that all nutritional supplements are taken with the consent of the conferring physician.

Nutrition

It is anticipated that with the right nutritional recommendation, the patient will be able to reach and sustain the best metabolic rates, thus controlling the blood glucose levels to a normal rage or at a minimum of an acceptable level.

These will assist the patient in avoiding or perhaps lessening the risk of other related complications that diabetes presents. The right nutrition regiment for diabetes is aimed to make sure a lipid and lipoprotein profile is sustained to lessen the risk of macrovascular disease.

The nutrition selection is also made to assist you in forming optimum blood pressure levels that would, in turn, assist you in lessen the risks of vascular diseases.

Nutrition regiments are also supposed to assist in preventing and treating chronic complications that occur in any diabetic patient. The nutritional recommendations are amended to guarantee an improved lifestyle so that the patient with diabetics can keep away from possible obesity, cardiovascular diseases, dyslipidemia, nephropathy, and hypertension. Taking the recommended nutrition would need the diabetic patient to have a sufficient amount of physical activity integrated with the lifestyle to ensure that there is no chance of the nutrient being preserved in the system and put together to result in more issues. You should take note that there are numerous different categories and levels of diabetic issues, and as a result, some cases may be different from the other. This means that any nutrition diet arrangement recommended has to be custom-fitted to the patient's requirements.

Diet Planning

A dietetic plan should make sure that all the carbohydrates are taken each diet every day is well spread out so as not to engulf the body system. This is vital as it assists in making sure that the blood sugar levels are kept in control. Therefore, there is the requirement to stay on the pathway of what is being eaten.

The number of carbs eaten can also be controlled while making use of insulin and performing exercise. The majority of the diabetic patent have to be worried about the sodium content of the foods they eat, as it is possible that it can play a negative part in the high blood pressure, which is presently in the majority of diabetic patients.

Those with an extra medical condition of hypertension would be conscious of taking in sodium. For diabetic patients with high levels of lipids while taking in saturated fats, cholesterol, and trans-fat would be watched.

While trying to create a meal plan for a diabetic patient, some basic points should be taken notice of. These might add to ensuring that the calories which are taking in are kept to about 10% to 20% coming from a protein source.

Meats, which include beef and chicken, should be thought about over other options. About 25% to 30% of the calories should emerge from fats. However, foods that have saturated and trans fats should either be eaten in bits or totally shun. About 50% to 60% of calories should emerge from carbohydrates. Taking in plenty of oranges and green vegetables will assist you to sustain the balance, they may include the likes of broccoli or carrots. Taking in sweet potatoes or brown rice is preferable rather than regular potatoes and white rice because it is more advisable to eat as it serves as a nutritional benefit.

Cutting the Sugar

For your breakfast options, which include cereal, try to add dried berries, cinnamon, apricots, or other kinds of dried fruits, which will assist it in leading to a naturally sweet flavor that would be the best option for a diabetic patient. Another method that you can use to cut out the sugar content is to use strawberry or homemade raspberry sauce on pancakes and waffles rather than the sweetened syrup.

If it is possible, try to replace sugar with fruit purees as they contain natural sugar and it is also one of the best options for a diabetic patient. This is most important when there are recipes that need the inclusion of one or more cups of sugar as the measurements for the ingredients.

When you want to prepare vegetable dishes, try to add some sweeter vegetables alongside strong-flavored vegetables as it will assist in sweetness and will be beneficial to the taste of the dish.

In that case, you will have to use a combination of ginger and carrots, mashed sweet potatoes with cinnamon, spinach with nutmeg, and other relevant combination which a person finds pleasing. When you buy pre-prepared food items, try to look for the food items that have the right labeling and will also permit the diabetic patient to make the right decisions and but the products that do not possess high sugar content. It is also possible to eliminate sugar if you try to cut it out little by little rather than all at once.

How to Heal Kidney Diseases with Dr. Sebi

Your kidneys are two organs that are about the size of your fist that are located near the bottom of your rib cage. Each kidney will be on either side of the spine. In each kidney, there are millions of tiny things called nephrons. These nephrons filter the blood.

You need your kidneys in order to have a healthy body. Your kidneys filter out all the impurities in the blood, excessive water, and waste products. All these toxins get stored in the bladder and then removes them through the urine. Your kidneys regulate the potassium, salt, and pH levels in your body. The kidneys also produce hormones that can control red blood cell production and helps regulate blood pressure. Your kidneys create a type of vitamin D that can help your body absorb calcium better.

Kidney disease will attack these nephrons. The damage it causes might leave the kidneys unable to get rid of the waste. There are about 26 million people in the United States who are affected by kidney disease. This happens when the kidneys get damaged and aren't able to function properly. This damage might be caused by different long-term chronic conditions, high blood pressure, and diabetes. Kidney disease could cause other problems such as malnutrition, nerve damage, and weak bones.

If it gets worse with time, the kidneys might completely stop working altogether. This means that you might have to undergo dialysis to help the kidneys perform. Dialysis is a medical treatment where a machine purifies and filters the blood. This won't cure the disease, but it does help prolong life.

Basically, any problem with your kidneys might lead to your blood not being purified well. This causes toxins to be accumulated in the blood. You might have a family history of kidney problems, high blood pressure, and diabetes. Recent studies show that overusing normal medications for various diseases can play a huge role in deteriorating the health of your kidneys. Many people are habitual users of medications, even for the slightest aches and pains. You have probably done it since you didn't know that these drugs could harm your health including your heart, liver, and kidneys. Many people today have moved to a more holistic approach for their health. Dr. Sebi knew what some scientists are trying to prove today. He might have known that people today would need his help in curing their kidney problems. Yes, he created a herbal remedy for kidney problems.

If you have been diagnosed with kidney disease, following Dr. Sebi's diet can help you. Make sure you talk with your doctor if you feel like something isn't quite right with your health. When you think about all the toxins being put into our bodies today, it isn't any wonder that there are so many people with kidney problems.

Dr. Sebi's kit combines many very healthy and rare herbs that he thought was perfect for any kidney problem. Unfortunately, not all problems can be treated with the same herbs. Dr. Sebi's kits let you customize them for your needs. Let's look at the ingredients:

UTI Special Mix

UTIs are the most common problem with kidneys. If you are constantly getting UTIs, this might help you stop getting them.

Kidney Stone Hunter

This herbal mix works against kidney stones. Even if you don't get kidney stones, this can help detoxify your body.

AHP Zinc Powder

AHP or ayurvedically herb purified zinc powder can be taken by anyone who has a zinc deficiency. Zinc deficiency can cause kidney problems.

Swarna Bang Tablets

This combination of herbs has been used for thousands of years to fight recurring UTIs. These are strong enough to help the kidneys, too.

Chandanadi Tablets

This herbal combination includes Daruharidra-Berberis aristata, sandalwood oil, karpoora, rala-shorearobusta, amalaki, acacia catechu, kattha, gandhabirojasatva, sugandhamaricha, and sandalwood. These herbs are combined in the correct proportion to get the perfect outcome.

Punarnava Special Kidney Mix

Some reports published about kidney disease claims panarnava is one herb that helps the kidneys function properly.

As you know, your kidneys are a critical filtration part of your body. Without it, we wouldn't be able to survive for long with all the toxins we are exposed to every day. Even the slightest of imbalances in filtering out toxins, we could be faced with problems like cysts, kidney stones, UTIs, gout, or other chronic and severe complications. Some are fairly common, but others can be life-threatening.

Dr. Sebi's kidney kit gives your body the minerals and herbs your body needs to keep your kidneys healthy. They can help your body function better by detoxifying your body. The herbs help to cleanse the kidneys of all the toxins it has stored up. This won't happen overnight; it will take several months for you to notice any results. Each kit will last for about two months.

When you go to Dr. Sebi's website, there will be some questionnaires for you to feel out. These will help them pick the right combination of herbs for you. You will then get to decide what you want to try in order to improve your health.

How to Heal Blood pressure with Dr. Sebi

When the pressure of your blood flow is higher than it should be when passing through the arteries and it consistently remains higher, then, you have high blood pressure. If your blood pressure happens to be 140/90, then taking steps to lower, it is the best chance you stand against the risk of kidney failure, stroke, heart attack, and other serious ailments.

A blood pressure gauge is only capable of registering two readings; the first and higher one is systolic while the second and lower one is diastolic. Diastolic pressure occurs before the heartbeats, and it is inaccurate for telling blood pressure. Systolic pressure, on the other hand, shows the pressure built up as the heart pumps blood out to the aorta, then the arteries. A high reading of systolic pressure shows the pathways have been altered either by hardened cell walls or plaques forming on in the arteries.

Clogging of the arteries brings about changes like hypertension which is usually caused by tobacco, stress, bad diet, aging, and overeating. High sodium intake, heredity, excessive coffee, and drug abuse are also likely causes of hypertension.

Dr. Sebi's recommended Herbs to Reduce High Blood Pressure

The herbs recommended by Dr. Sebi for the treatment of blood pressure include the following;

- Black cohosh
- Chamomile
- Yellow dock
- Oregano
- Fennel
- Saffron
- Valerian root
- Basil
- Hawthorne berries widen blood vessels and coronary arteries.
- Cayenne

How Does 'The Doctor Sebi Alkaline Diet' Prevent Hypertension?

Dr. Sebi High blood pressure medication (natural herbs):

The doctor recommends the following herbs since they open the walls of the arteries, open blood vessels, and remove plaques from the artery walls. The herbs have a high concentration of minerals and also contain natural alkaline. They have been certified as medications effective for dealing with high blood pressure. These herbs have high amounts of iron. They are: Cayenne, oregano, basil, black cohosh, fennel, yellow dock

Every drug used for high blood pressure in markets acts like water

Therefore, people must drink plenty of water. Divide your weight by half then consume that amount of water on a daily basis.

Eating five various types of vegetables and fruits every day will help in preventing clogging of the arteries due to a lot of plaque deposits

Vegetables and fruits have a higher level of antioxidants. Fruits and vegetables that contain a high percentage of antioxidants assist in protecting the arteries from the deposits. Examples of vegetables and fruits include oranges, cabbages, tomatoes, peaches, and seeded grapes.

Foods rich in potassium assist in reducing the recurrent high blood pressure since it removes the excess amounts of sodium from our bodies

A good example is red potatoes.

Fruits that contain fiber also have an impact on high blood pressure

The foods lower the blood pressure by eliminating waste products from the walls of the arteries.

High blood pressure after eating:

Knowledge in foods to eat related to high blood pressure is vital. You do not want to obtain high blood pressure as a result of eating similar foods to any other person. Below is a list of foods that you can avoid:

- You should avoid overeating even if the food is healthy.
- You should also avoid salty foods. Salty foods turn to plaques on the walls of the arteries. In general, you should avoid sodas, meat tenderizers, soy sauce, and baking soda.
- Hardly consume canned foods.
- Do away with dairy products like; cheese, alcohol, and sodium from your meal.
- You should not eat during evening hours.
- You should avoid all types of rice except the brown and wild ones.

Healing and Recovering from STDs with Dr. Sebi

STDs, which stands for sexually transmitted diseases, are still fairly prevalent even though there are well-known ways to prevent them. There are several diseases that fall into the category of STDs and are spread by sexual intercourse but can be spread through other manners. The most common STDs are trichomoniasis, syphilis, some types of hepatitis, gonorrhea, genital warts, genital herpes, Chlamydia, and HIV.

At one time, STDs were referred to as venereal diseases. They are some of the most common contagious infections. About 65 million Americans have been diagnosed with an incurable STD. Every year, 20 million new cases occur, and about half of these are in people aged 15 to 24. All of these can have long-term implications.

These are serious illnesses that need to be treated. Some of them are considered incurable and can be deadly, such as HIV. Learning more about these diseases can provide you with knowledge on how to protect yourself.

STDs can be spread through oral, vaginal, and anal sex. Trichomoniasis is able to be contracted through contact with a moist or damp object, like toilet seats, wet clothing, or towels, although it is mostly spread through sexual contact. People who are at a higher risk of STDs include:

- Those who have more than one sexual partner.
- Those who trade sex for drugs or money.
- Those who share needles for drug use.
- Those who don't use condoms during sex.
- Those who have sex with a person who has had several partners.

Herpes and HIV are the two STDs that are chronic conditions that modern medicine cannot cure, but can only manage. Hepatitis B can sometimes become chronic. Unfortunately, you sometimes don't find out that you have an STD until it has damaged your reproductive organs, heart, vision, or other organs. STDs can also weaken the immune system, which leaves you vulnerable to contracting other diseases. Chlamydia and gonorrhea can cause pelvic inflammatory disease, and this can leave women unable to conceive. It is also able to kill you. If an STD is passed onto a newborn, the baby could face permanent damage, or it could kill them.

Causes of STDs

In terms of modern medicine, STDs are caused by all types of infection. Syphilis, gonorrhea, and Chlamydia are bacteria. Hepatitis B, genital warts, genital herpes, and HIV are all viral. Parasites cause trichomoniasis.

The STD germs live within vaginal secretions, blood semen, and, in some cases, saliva. The majority of the organisms will be spread through oral, anal, or vaginal sex, but some, like with genital warts and genital herpes, can be spread simply through skin-to-skin contact. Hepatitis B is able to be spread through sharing personal items, like razors or toothbrushes.

Prevention

The most obvious step in healing for STDs is to not get one in the first place. The first tip people give in preventing STDs is to not have sex, or at least avoid sex with people who have genital discharge, rash, sores, or other symptoms. The only time you should have unprotected sex is if you and your partner are only having sex with one another, and you have both tests negative for STDs in the last six months. Otherwise, you need to make sure you:

Use condoms whenever you have sex. If you need a lubricant, make sure that it is one that is water-based. Condoms should be used for the entire act of sex. Keep in mind; condoms aren't 100% effective when it comes to preventing pregnancy or disease. However, they are very effective if you use them the right way.

Avoid sharing underclothing or towels.

Bathe after and before you have sex.

If you are okay with vaccination, you can get vaccines for a lot of STDs, specifically Hep B and HPV.

Make sure you are tested for HIV.

If you abuse alcohol or drugs, please seek help. It is more common for people who are under the influence to have unsafe sex.

Lastly, abstaining from sex completely is the only 100% effective way to prevent STDs.

There was a time when it was believed that using a condom with nonoxynol-9 would prevent STDs by killing the organisms that caused them. There has been new research that has found that this can end up irritating the woman's cervix and vagina and could increase her risk of an STD. It is recommended that you avoid condoms with nonoxynol-9.

How to Heal Herpes with Dr. Sebi

The most common symptoms of herpes are vaginal discharge, cold sores, pain during urination, ulcers, and blisters. There is modern medicine that can help with herpes, but none of them can cure it.

There are two forms of the HSV virus: simplex one and two. Simplex one is considered oral herpes, and simplex two is genital herpes. Over 50% of the people in the US have simplex one. In the US, about 15.5% of people aged 14 to 49 have simplex two.

If you receive oral sex from a person who has a current outbreak of cold sores around the mount ups your risk of being infected. You cannot contract genital herpes from a toilet seat.

The majority of people who have been infected with herpes won't experience any symptoms for months or years. Those who do end up having an outbreak during this initial period will have it within four days of exposure, but it can range from two to 12 days.

Most people who are infected with HSV will have recurring outbreaks. When a person has first been infected with herpes, they will have recurrences more frequently. With time, though, the remission phases will get longer, and recurrences won't be as severe.

The primary infection is the outbreak of genital herpes that happens after a person has just been infected. The symptoms of the first outbreak tend to be very severe and could involve:

- Red blisters on the skin
- Cold sores on or around the mouth
- Malaise
- High temperature

- Pain during urination
- Enlarged, tender lymph nodes
- Itching and pain
- Vaginal discharge
- Ulceration and blisters on the external genitalia, on the cervix, or in the vagina

Most of the time, those sores will heal up, and there won't be any noticeable scarring. In outbreaks after the primary outbreak, the symptoms aren't as severe and don't last as long. Most of the time, symptoms don't last longer than ten days and will often include:

- Red blisters
- Cold sores on or around the mouth
- Women could have ulcers or blisters on the cervix
- Tingling or burning around the genitals before the blisters show up

If HSV is present on the skin of a person infected with it, it can be given to another person through the moist skin in the genitals, anus, and mouth. The virus can also spread to other people through contact with other areas of the skin, including the eyes.

You cannot catch HSV by touching a towel, sink, work surface, or object that was touched by the infected person. An infection will most often occur in one of the following ways:

- Having genital contact with a person who is infected.
- Sharing sex toys.
- Having oral sex with a person with current cold sores.
- Having unprotected anal or vaginal sex.

It is most common for the virus to be passed on right before the blisters appear, while visible, and until the blisters have completely gone away. HSV is also able to be passed on to another person even if there aren't any signs of a current outbreak, but it isn't that likely.

It is possible for a baby to get herpes from its mother if she has an active outbreak at the time she gives birth.

As far as modern medicine goes, there are various treatment options, most of which are home remedies. Home remedies for herpes include:

- Painkillers, like ibuprofen or acetaminophen
- Bathing in an Epsom salt bath to help relieve symptoms
- Soaking in a sitz bath
- Using petroleum jelly on the affected skin
- Avoiding tight clothing
- Washing hands well, especially when you have touched an affected area

- Abstaining from sex until the symptoms have past
- If urinating hurts, rub some lidocaine lotion or cream to the urethra
- There are some people who like to apply ice packs to the affected area.

There aren't any drugs that can get rid of herpes. Doctors will sometimes prescribe antivirals, like acyclovir, which can help prevent the virus from spreading. They can also help an outbreak to clear up quicker and can help to reduce symptom severity.

Doctors will normally only prescribe antivirals the first time a person has an outbreak. Subsequent outbreaks tend to be mild, so treatment isn't normally needed.

There is also an episodic treatment option, which is used on people who have less than six outbreaks in a single year. Whenever an outbreak occurs, a doctor will prescribe a five-day course of antivirals.

If a person has more than six outbreaks in a single year, a doctor may prescribe a suppressive treatment. There are some cases where a doctor could recommend that a person takes an antiviral each day for the rest of your life. The point of this is to try and prevent any more outbreaks. While this suppressive treatment is able to significantly reduce your risk of passing herpes onto your partner, there is still a small chance that you can.

To prevent herpes, you should follow the same prevent rules that were listed above, plus avoid kissing anybody if they have a cold sore. For most people, there are types of triggers that will cause an outbreak. These triggers could be sunbathing, friction against the skin, illness, being tired, and stress. Figuring out triggers can help to lower a person's chance of an outbreak.

Now, you can do the above, or you can try Dr. Sebi's cure. The goal of following Dr. Sebi's treatment is to create an environment where herpes can't live. Cells need to receive oxygen. Then chemicals in regular medications for herpes remove oxygen from and cells, and most of the time, will also introduce herpes. It will take some time to help cleanse your body of herpes, but you'll do it with iron-rich plant-based items. You should start out by taking Bio Ferro and Iron Plus. Then you will need to start eating foods high in iron, which include:

- Yellow dock
- Blue vervain
- Burdock
- Lams quarters
- Dandelion

- Kale
- Purslane
- Conconsa
- Guaco
- Sarsil berry
- Sarsaparilla

Then you will want to have some bromide plus powder. The iron you are consuming is boosting your immune system, but you need to get mineral nutrition, and that's where the bromide plus powder comes in. All you have to do for this is to mix a teaspoon into a cup of boiling water. You should consume this at least two times a day.

More important than what you should consume is what you shouldn't consume. It is important that you avoid sweets and starches. You can have small amounts of sweet plant food or fruits. It is best to choose bitter foods rather than sweet. When it comes to herpes, you will want to stay away from quinoa, avocados, and chickpeas, and try to consume cactus plants, mushrooms, squash, and zucchini, as well as sea vegetables.

You can make teas out of plants like yellow dock, dandelion, and burdock. These should be consumed several times throughout the day for at least ten days. Depending on where you live, you may have to order these herbs online. You should also practice fasting. The more you are able to faster, the quicker your body will heal from herpes. If, while fasting, you start to feel weak, you can eat some dates. They may be sweet, but they won't affect your cells. Make sure you only eat them if you feel weak.

You should also eat plenty of salads. As a rule of thumb, eat salad as if you were eating a bag of potato chips, but don't eat iceberg.

Chapter 4: Dr. Sebi Fasting

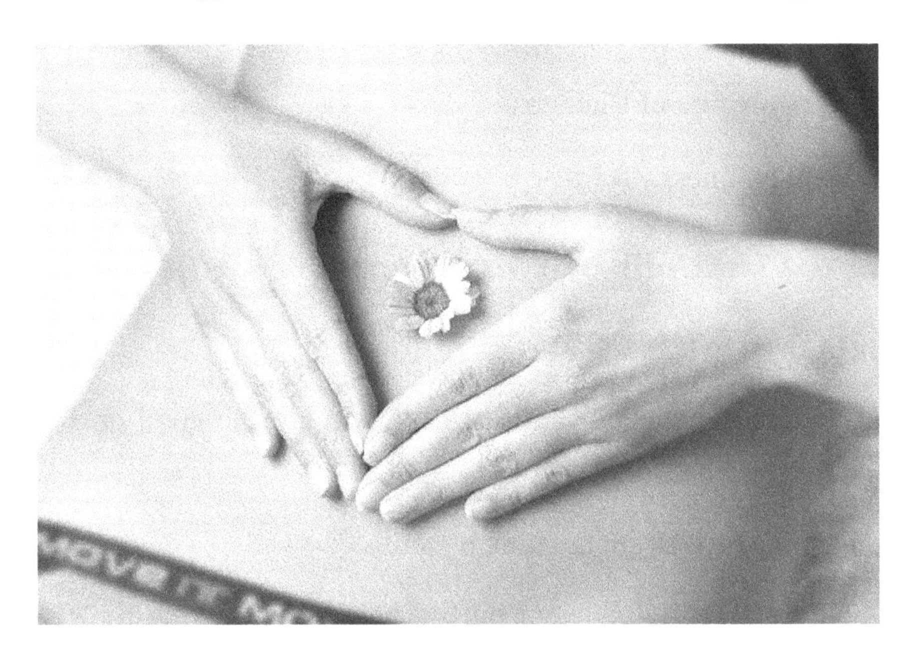

The power of fasting the Dr. Sebi way: what fasting did for Dr. Sebi

1. It healed him of his diabetes.

2. He cured him of impotence.

3. He was able to satisfy his wife in bed.

When you practice fasting the Dr. Sebi way, here are the benefits you will get:

- Detoxifying of your body.
- Healing of your body.

- Restoration of health and vitality.
- Cure you of impotence.
- Cure you of Diabetes.
- Freshness.

Eight facts about Dr. Sebi's fasting life

1. He loved to fast.

2. He firmly believed that fasting made him be good on the bed for his wife.

3. Fasting gave Dr. Sebi many benefits.

4. He taught his followers on the benefits of fasting the Dr. Sebi way.

5. He explained that every Dr. Sebi follower should fast 12 days every year.

6. He fasted for more than 90 days.

7. His diabetes was cured after 30 days of fasting.

8. His impotence was healed after 52 days of fasting.

How to fast the way Dr. Sebi approved way

Time of fasting should be happy moments for you. You should always be happy when you begin a fasting journey.

Fasting Dr. Sebi's way will mean that you are taking after the footsteps of Dr. Sebi and doing precisely what he has taught his followers as regards fasting.

Fasting has been a common practice among many individuals in the world. The Muslims do fast, likewise the Christians. But the way of fasting, as done by the Muslims and Christians is not the same as that of Dr. Sebi.

The Dr. Sebi fasting method is a unique one. Beyond its uniqueness, it is also easy to practice. It is a major way of detoxifying your body. So, if you want to live healthily and regain all your lost vitality, then Fasting the Dr. Sebi way is the only and right method to adopt.

How to begin fasting the Dr. Sebi Approved way

You cannot begin on a fasting exercise without preparation. You cannot even try that of adopting the Dr. Sebi fasting method. It is dangerous!

Your body will need a great measure of nutrition. Hence, you need to start preparing as early as possible. Dr. Sebi recommended that you take a minimum of 1 week to begin your preparation.

You can likewise use two or three weeks in preparing for fasting the Dr. Sebi way. What you should do:

1. The first step to take is to commence eating alkaline electric diets.

2. Get your herbs and supplies ready. It will be hard for you to do the Dr. Sebi fasting method without herbs. I tried it without herbs for 12 days, and it was tough on me. Ensure you stock your kitchen with enough of the Dr. Sebi recommended herbs.

What you need when fasting the Dr. Sebi way.

Lots of water and juice: This is very important in staying hydrated. During Dr. Sebi's fasting schedules, he drank lots of water and juice.

It is recommended you don't run short of water and juice during Dr. Sebi's fasting schedule. Dr. Sebi drank the Tamarind juice, but you can also take any other juice as they are okay and approved by Dr. Sebi.

You can check Dr. Sebi approved **juice list** here or check through the other books authored by me. Take a half cup glass of juice.

Three capsules of Green food pl.us. The green food plus contains the following:

(i) Linden leaf

(ii) Bladderwrack

(iii) Nopal

(iv) Stinging Nettles

Sea Moss Tea: Dr. Sebi also drank sea moss tea during his fasting schedules. You should also prepare your sea moss tea and take it during your fasting period.

Fasting is the beginning of life.

Now you are ready. After you have made all ready and you are waiting for your fasting schedule, what you are expected to do is to rest and relax.

On day 1, you will have to adjust to your fast. Since you have chosen to go fasting the Dr. Sebi way, it is a must you follow all Dr. Sebi approved steps.

On the first day, you will take 3 cups of green food plus. Also, take as much water and juice as you want.

This should be done in the morning. But ensure you don't gorge yourself on liquids. Drink a lot of water to your desire and satisfaction.

Also, take spring water. But if you don't have readily available, you can easily add lime to your water. Please, stay away from tap water.

What you should expect

1. You will go through many stages.

2. Usually, the first 3 days of your fasting are the toughest.

3. You will be hungry the first day and tempted not to continue.

4. You can take a half glass cup of juice to sleep easily when you are hungry.

5. Day 2 will be easier, and the third day will go fast.

6. By day 5, you are almost familiar with the schedule. So, you won't be hungry anymore.

7. On day 9, you will see mucus in your stool. This should make you happy.

8. You should expect to fall sick and nauseated between days 6 and 14.

9. After day 10, your brain becomes clearer. Parasites might also come out from your stool.

10. You will feel better and happier on day 10 as insomnia will fade away.

What should you expect?

The stages involved in your fasting journey are many. The first three days of your fasting are the most difficult. The very first day will get you into a famished and unsure state about how to complete the day. When this feeling creeps in, take half a cup of diluted or undiluted fruit to help you get some sleep. Things will get a tad bit easier on the 2nd day, and by the 3rd day, your body is already adjusting to your new lifestyle.

By day 5, you won't feel any hunger in you, and on the 9th day, mucus will be in your stool.

Between days 6 to 14, you can expect to be nauseous and sick. Dr. Sebi's first fasting experience was no different and one woman who happened to fast in that same period to cure her diabetes said: "prepare to be sick."

On day 10, your brain will become clearer than it has possibly been and the parasites in your body will be purged through your stool. Your insomnia will be gone, and you will be happy.

After the first two weeks, you must be prepared for everything that is to come. You will be angry and frustrated. To top it all, your brain will play back memories that had been buried deep in you; some of these memories might scare you.

When you are in danger

You might be in danger and not know it.

If you happen to visit the bathroom less than two times a day, you need to start taking Sagrada, laxatives, or some other alternatives that can help you loosen your stool. Parsley and Burdock tea are great natural alternatives to chemical medicinal solutions.

It may happen that a dead parasite is blocking your colon. This can lead to vomiting, and when this happens, all you need to do is get a pineapple and make a juice out of it. This juice must drink at once to help move the parasitic blockage in your colon.

A vast majority of people who partake in this fasting journey do have a buttery smooth ride. However, if you happen to be among the few who experience a breakout on their skin a few days after starting the fast, it is advised that you stop totally as the toxins in your body are being excreted from the skin instead of your urine and stool.

Weakness, passing out, and inability to walk might creep in while you are fasting. When this happens, it is advised that you take a day or two off to get back on track, and once you feel better than before, you can continue on with your fasting journey. If you can make it past a week on this fasting diet, then, you really have a strong will. With this fasting method, anger, frustration, and venting have been recorded due to partakers no having a taste of their favorite food or any food at all.

Once you get past this anger and frustration phase then, you can move on to what the future holds – a diet with no junk food.

Life is not a bed of roses, but we all hope to live long, healthy, and happy. Tomorrow will be better, but today we have to rest and count our blessings. In the end, all the struggles will be worth it with a little happiness in our minds.

Dr. Sebi intermittent fasting diet

Prayer and intermittent fasting diet can be made into a cycle of renewal for your body, spirit, and mind. Fasting is a diet that cleanses the body. The spiritual, physical, and mental are all put to rest. Your abstinence, restraint, and self-discipline come into play on how well your body will use its skills to purge wastes, impurities, and excess mucus which does nothing but degenerate the health and lead to ill-health. Regeneration and healing of the organs also go on behind the scenes.

Fasting is an easy exercise, but it is not something for the faint-hearted individual. Fasting without proper guidance will have an individual confused about why it seems like depression is setting in, dreams of sumptuous meals creep in, it looks like you are starving yourself for nothing, and nausea is setting in. A faint-hearted individual will find solace in all the food they gave up for a healthy lifestyle – back to square one.

If you know the right places to look, you will find a lot of information about how fasting benefits the body tremendously in terms of natural healing, cleansing, and the best ways to fast. Contained on this page is the best discovery on intermittent fasting that will change your life forever.

How fasting heals the body

Fasting has been in vogue for years because it was discovered that during this period of intentionally staying away from food, the body rids itself of cells and tissues that aid diseases. A thorough general cleansing process also goes on in the body. Fasting is a way of giving your body the go-ahead to use its natural capacity to self-heal.

When you start fasting, you are not just depriving yourself of food; you are sending a message to your body that it is time for them to activate their eliminative ability. When all the organs receive this message in the body, the skin, liver, lungs, and kidney start to expel a massive amount of waste, toxin, and mucus out of the body.

The better your approach to fasting, the better your chances of efficiently expelling waste and toxins. Even better is your state of health.

To properly cleanse the body during a fasting period, it is advised to ingest water, raw juices, vegetable juices soups, and broths only. You just have to know what you want and go for the kind of fasting that best suits your needs.

Dr. Sebi's cleanse to heal the body

According to Dr. Sebi, fasting heals the body in a number of ways unimaginable. Vegetable soups and raw juices are considered as the best consumables during fasting because they are rich in vitamins, minerals, enzymes, and trace elements. These properties complement the body, and they are easily absorbed without the body exhausting the energy it's meant to use for healing on food digestion.

Benefits of juice fasting

The significance of vegetable and fruit juices can never be underplayed as their nutritious elements help the body to regenerate cells quickly and speed up healing activities. Again, Dr. Sebi's ailments only disappeared after he had fasted for 90 days.

Fasting on vegetables both and raw juices

Raw juices and broth maintain a perfect balance of the blood and tissues in the body. According to Dr. Sebi, fasting increases the number of acids the blood and the tissues have. Vegetable juices from raw fruits and broth provide the body with more-than-enough alkaline liquid to restore tissues and cells and also to create a balance in the PH levels. The biological chemical structure of the body gets balanced with the help of the minerals from juices and broths.

Fasting benefits of juices, vegetables, and water

The high mineral elements contained in raw and vegetable juices is why they are preferred over water during fasting.

Asides that, they help to neutralize DDT, poisons, and other toxins contained in the bloodstream.

Overall, vegetable/juice fasting is favored over water fasting for apparent reasons. The former will increase your body's ability to eliminate and detoxify apparatus, and the healing journey will be quicker than using water.

Simple Rules of Starting:

Adapting to the fasting schedule takes time.

Start with a short period of fasting, and you can fast longer as time goes by.

Avoid calories during the fast.

Avoid extreme workouts while fasting. On days you know you want your workout to the extreme, avoid fasting that day.

Avoid rushing your food. Do not overeat. Eat slowly to help your body digest better. Spread your meals throughout your feeding window.

Do away with junk foods and poor eating habits. Opt for nutrient-dense high-quality foods instead.

Keep your body hydrated by drinking a lot of water.

Chapter 5: Weight Reduction in a Healthy Manner

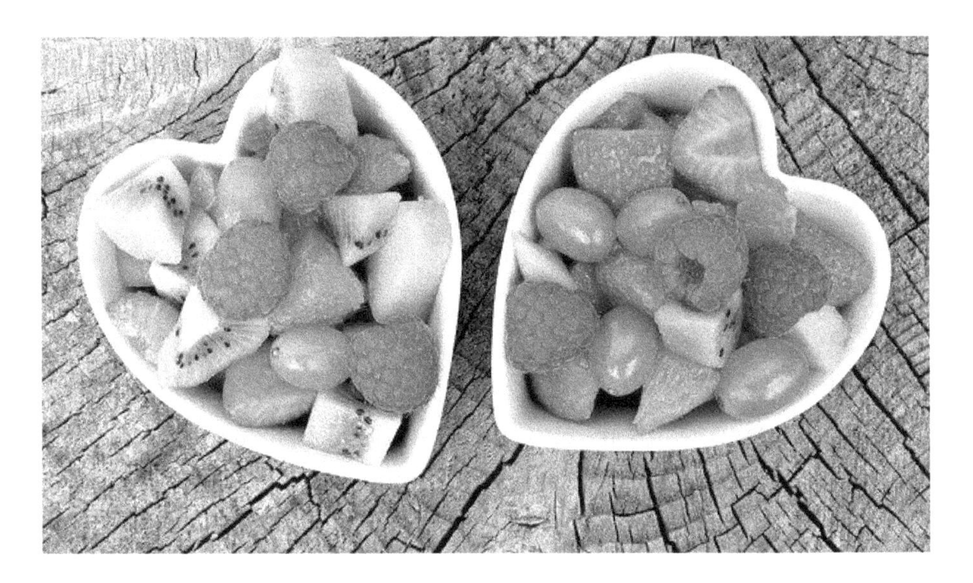

The Dr. Sebi diet is often referred to as the African biomineral balance. This was how he would cure people of a variety of diseases. It is basically a vegan diet that is made up of foods that he called "electric" or alkaline foods. It is suggested that, while following this diet, you also take his healing supplements.

You cannot eat any meat or animal products while on this diet, as well as foods that contain a lot of starch. The reason for this is that you are only supposed to eat alkaline-forming foods, and those foods form acids.

Meat products cause uric acid production, dairy produces cause lactic acid, and starch causes carbonic acid. All of these acids will build up, which causes a buildup of mucus. The mucus robs our cells of oxygen. However, if you eat electric foods, they feed the body. The human body is electrical, so it needs electric food to function.

This diet is made up of grains, teas, nuts, veggies, and fruits. Among the foods you can eat are wild rice, amaranth, quinoa, mushrooms, watercress, kale, dates, figs, mangos, avocados, and much more. These foods will help to nourish your body and won't end up causing an accumulation of mucus.

If you plan on really starting this diet, you must make sure that you really want it. The first thing you will need to do is to make some changes to how you eat. You will probably find that this is going to require you to be your best emotional state and the right state of mind.

Eating is a big part of our life, and the types of things we consume form strong habits that can end up lasting our entire life. It can be very hard to break these habits and deal with the influence of family and friends. That means, before you jump right into this diet, you should take some time thinking about changing how you eat. You don't want to promise yourself this and then end up not being able to follow through just because you weren't prepared.

Instead, you should begin slowly. You can even talk to your family and friends. The reaction you can get from people when you talk to them about Dr. Sebi's diet will vary. Some will want to learn more, while others will write it off as bunk.

That being said, you shouldn't tire yourself by trying to convince everybody else before you make sure that it is right for you. Your vitality, health improvements, and cleaner outlook will show your family way more than just your words.

Once you do start making the transition, the first thing you need to do is to start reading food ingredient labels on everything. This will help you to stay conscious about what you are drinking and eating. When you are first starting out, before you live completely by the nutritional guide, this awareness is going to provide you with the incentive to change things as you continue on. Later on, if you do end up straying from the diet, you will still be able to remain conscious about what you are eating.

If you have long been a meat-eater, that may be the hardest thing to transition from. The best thing you can do is to start making the transition from meats by switching to eating only fish. Then you can slowly start eating less and less fish each week.

It is also important that you start making your own snacks. This will ensure if you do get the urge to snack, that you will have good snacks to eat. Approved nuts and raisins are a good choice.

Then you need to make sure that you are eating all of the correct foods. That means you need to learn what foods are and aren't on the nutritional guide. You must stick to only those foods. At first, this will feel tough, and that is expected. In fact, it is very hard to do in our society when only the bad foods are pushed at us. This is the reason why I stressed that you must be emotionally ready.

You also need to make sure you are drinking plenty of water. While we have all known for a while now that water is a very important part of our health, most of us are still not drink enough. Plus, there are a lot of Dr. Sebi products that you will be taking, like the Bromide Plus Powder, contain herbs that act as diuretics. That means you have to take extra care to make sure you don't allow yourself to get dehydrated.

Dr. Sebi suggests that you drink a gallon of spring water every day. Springwater has a natural alkaline pH, whereas tap water can be high in chloride and many other contaminants.

You will also need to learn how to cook your own meals if you don't cook already. You aren't going to find too many prepackaged foods that fit into the Dr. Sebi diet. Once you do get the hang of cooking, you will find that you can change your favorite dishes into Dr. Sebi-approved dishes.

The Best Way to Balance Your Body

The acid-alkaline diet comes in various names. You may be confounded when you hear them. In any case, recall that they all relate to a specific something - knowing the nourishments that structure acid and those that structure alkaline side-effect. A portion of the well-known names is alkaline debris diet and alkaline acid diet. In light of the guideline of the arrangement, nourishments are characterized into three: acid, alkaline, or impartial. The response is controlled by knowing its answer with water.

Your diet is the essential motivation behind why you endure all the crippling diseases that are already obscure. Early individuals are eating, for the most part, products of the soil and almost no prepared nourishments. Yet, with the cutting-edge innovation and quick-paced way of life, more individuals are including meat and handled items into their diet. These nourishment items are acid makers. As per the defenders of the acid-alkaline food, you should take nourishments that incorporate increasingly alkaline details rather than acid. This is because the blood is principally alkaline. It has a pH of 7.35 to 7.45. In light of their contentions, you need to keep up this normal pH to advance the most extreme health. This is because essential supplements are better caught up with a somewhat alkaline body liquid.

An acid-alkaline diet gives a few health benefits. Besides the undeniable preferred position of keeping the pH parity of the body, it can assist rule with the trip a few diseases, including diabetes, cancer, and gastric issues. Different indications that can be precluded incorporate the accompanying:

- Loss of energy
- Nasal blockage
- Anxiety and apprehension
- Headache

If you need to pursue the acid-alkaline diet, specialists guide you to take more leafy foods rather than meat, salt, and handled nourishments. These acid-delivering nourishments are the reasons why you experience the ill effects of various health issues.

Before you start with the acid-alkaline diet, you should initially counsel your primary care physician. Try not to take this sort of food on the off chance that you have kidney issues. This can just intensify your condition. You should likewise work intimately with your health care specialist on the off chance that you have previous health issues.

This is a major one, for who hasn't had a weight issue at once or another? Furthermore, for the individuals who have, what might you have given for a straightforward, sheltered, and free approach to getting more fit?

The regular western diet and way of life are made out of such a large number of acid-creating substances (refined flours, sugars, meat, and dairy items) and propensities (smoking, liquor utilization, and physician endorsed drug use) that our bodies have gotten immersed with acid squanders. What's more, acids have an awful method for eating into and breaking down healthy muscle, tissues, and even organs.

One of the programmed guard instruments of the body is to deliver fat cells to shield our sensitive organs from these overabundance acids. The fat cells' capacity is to carry these acid squanders away from the organs and store it in less significant pieces of the body, however, as long as there are abundant acids in the body, the fat cells will stick to the organs protectively. When we can free ourselves of these abundance acids (through keeping up a high-alkaline diet, legitimate hydration, and exercise), the fat cells are never again required, and the body discharges them from obligation, bringing about weight loss.

Dr. Sebi Diet Weight Loss

This part is clear as crystal. Weight loss will undoubtedly happen when following the diet because the Dr. Sebi diet comprises of common vegetables, organic products, grains, nuts, and vegetables. It disposes of waste, dairy, meat, and handled nourishment, so usually, you will shed pounds. The

Dr. Sebi diet fills in as a cleanser and receives numerous rewards, including your body expressing gratitude toward you.

The Dr. Sebi diet advances eating entire, natural, plant-based nourishment. It might help weight loss on the off chance that you don't typically eat like this. Nonetheless, it intensely depends on taking the maker's costly enhancements, is exceptionally prohibitive, does not have certain supplements, and mistakenly vows to change your body to an alkaline state. In case you're hoping to pursue a more plant-based eating design, numerous healthy diets are progressively adaptable and practical.

Imagine a scenario in which you thought about a weight loss program that would assist you with getting in shape and feel more youthful. OK, attempt it? The alkaline diet and way of life have been around for more than 60 years, yet numerous individuals aren't acquainted with its regular, protected, and demonstrated weight loss properties!

The alkaline diet isn't a contrivance or a prevailing fashion. It's a healthy and straightforward approach to appreciate new degrees of health. In this post, you'll find out about what this dietary arrangement is, the thing that makes it unique, and how it can create groundbreaking outcomes for you, your waistline, and your health. It is right to say that you are getting a charge out of a thin and attractive body today? Assuming this is the case, you're in the minority.

Unfortunately, more than 65 percent of Americans are either overweight or hefty. In case you're overweight, you presumably experience indications of ill health like weakness, expanding, sore joints, and a large group of different signs of unexpected frailty. More terrible yet, you most likely want to abandon regularly getting a charge out of the body you need and merit. Maybe you've been informed that you're merely getting more established, yet that isn't necessarily reality. Try not to get tied up with that falsehood. Different societies have healthy, lean seniors who appreciate excellent health into their nineties!

Indeed, your body is a splendidly planned machine, and on the off chance that you have any side effects of ill health, this is a sure sign that your body's science is excessively acidic. Your side effects are only a weep for help. This is because the body doesn't merely separate one day. Slightly, your health disintegrates gradually after some time, at last falling into 'disease.'

Acid to Alkaline Diet, How to Lose Weight and Live a Healthier Lifestyle Naturally

Acid to Alkaline Diet

The acid to alkaline diet is turning into a more discussed subject these days, yet at the same time, most of the populace are unconscious of what it is. Individuals who bite the dust youthful, have health issues, experience the ill effects of heftiness and so on., by and large, have an extremely acidic inside condition though individuals who live to mature age and don't experience the ill effects of genuine health issues have an interior situation that is increasingly alkaline.

In the cutting-edge Western world by far, most of the individuals carry on with an unhealthy way of life, overwhelmingly eating garbage and unhealthy nourishment and being always presented to different variables that drastically negatively sway our health, in drastic differentiation to the acid to an alkaline diet. As per the World Health Organization (WHO), there are more than one billion overweight grown-ups around the world, with around 300 million of them clinically fat. This measurement is unnerving and is dramatically expanding ordinary!

Then again, if an individual's body is too acidic they can without much of a stretch encounter weight by picking up and clutching fat, they will age snappier, an absence of energy will be healthy, they will effectively and reliably draw in disease and infection's and make an inside situation where yeast and microorganisms can undoubtedly flourish.

Most of the individuals living in the Western world don't pursue an acid to an alkaline diet and are commonly more on the acidic scale. This is generally expected in our menu. Eating things like shoddy nourishment, burgers, bubbly drinks, having a high sugar consumption, singed food sources, unnatural organic product juices, impersonation nourishments, energy drinks, and prepared food sources, for instance, all push our bodies inside condition down on the acidic scale. There are even some generally healthy nourishments to know about, strawberries, mangos, and peaches, for instance, are high in sugar, in this manner make an acidic situation in the body. Some different astonishments that likewise cause acidic to develop incorporate rice, fish, oats, and cheddar, so these nourishments are to be constrained when following an acid to an alkaline diet. This is one motivation behind why it is essential to know what nourishments will cause an acid response and which will make you increasingly salty. Different contemplations that likewise cause our bodies to be increasingly acidic incorporate various synthetics, tobacco, radiation, pesticides, fake sugars, air contamination, liquor, drugs, and stress.

The ideal pH to get every one of the advantages of alkalinity is 7.4pH. If your body goes, 3-4 focuses whichever way you will pass on! The pH scale is as per the following:

0 = complete acid/sulfuric acid, hydrochloric acid

1 = gastric juices

2 = vinegar

3 = lager

4 = wine, tomato juice

5 = downpour

6 = milk

7 = unadulterated water

8 = ocean water

9 = preparing pop

10 = cleanser, milk of magnesia

11 = alkali, lime water

12 = dye

13 = lye

14 = Total Alkaline/Sodium Hydroxide

The acid to the alkaline diet will enable your body to remain at the ideal range, around 7.4pH. The body's response to attempting to keep this acid, alkaline parity, is both fantastic and exciting. At the point when your body is too acidic, it has a go at everything to get to an increasingly alkaline state. At the position when this happens, the body stores some acid in your fat to prevent it from doing damage to our body, which is something to be thankful for, yet your body at that point clutches the fat for security, making the individual put on weight. When there is an abundance of acid inside, the body finds alkaline somewhere else from your bones and teeth, yet your bones and teeth get so drained that they become delicate and begin to rot. This can prompt numerous diseases of the bones and teeth, including joint inflammation and tooth rot. This would not occur if an individual were following an acid to an alkaline diet.

The development of acid, for the most part, will settle away from your healthier organs; however, instead, it floats towards your weakest organs that are as of now inclined to disease. It resembles a pack of wolves searching for the lowest among the group, taking out the simple prey. As your flimsier organs are focused on, it makes it a lot simpler for certain diseases to set in, including cancer. Realize that cancer cells become lethargic on the off chance that you are at 7.4pH (which is the body's ideal pH levels), therefore further underlining the significance of keeping up a healthy pH level in our bodies by following the acid to an alkaline diet. When there is acid in the framework, it additionally taints your circulatory system. This like this forestalls the types of blood capacity to deliver oxygen to the tissues. RBC's are encompassed by a negative charge so they can skip off one another and move around in the blood rapidly and give their decency.

However, when you are too acidic, they lose their negative charge, and they remain together, making them move gradually. This makes them battle to deliver supplements and oxygen in our framework. One of the primary manifestations of this harming is you begin to feel a loss of energy even though you are getting enough rest. Beginning an acid to the alkaline diet can address this rapidly. Your blood likewise has this response in the wake of drinking liquor. We should place this into point of view; it takes around 33 glasses of water to kill one glass of coke! I'm not, in any case, going to refer to the stuff to destroy a portion of different things that we are placing into our bodies, I think you get the image!

What's going on with how you're eating now?

I'm sure you're acquainted with the term pH, which alludes to the degree of acidity or alkalinity contained in something. Alkalinity is estimated on a scale. You can take a necessary and reasonable test at home to see where your alkalinity level falls, just as to screen it routinely.

Medical analysts and researchers have known for in any event 70 years this lesser-known fact. Your body requires a specific pH level, or sensitive parity of your body's acid-alkaline levels - for ideal health and imperativeness.

You may think..."I don't have to know this science. Besides, what does the best possible pH parity and alkalinity matter to me?" I know these were my inquiries when I initially found out about alkaline eating.

We'll utilize two instances of how acid and alkalinity assume a job in your body.

1. We, as a whole, realize that our stomach has acid in it. Alongside proteins, this acid is fundamental for breaking nourishment into essential components that can be consumed by the stomach related tract. Consider the possibility that we didn't have any acid in our stomachs. We would kick the bucket from lack of healthy sustenance right away because the body couldn't use an entire bit of meat or a whole bit of anything, so far as that is concerned! Bode well?

2: Different pieces of our body require various degrees of acidity or alkalinity. For instance, your blood requires a somewhat more alkaline level than your stomach acids. Consider the possibility that your blood was excessively acidic. It would eat through your veins and conduits, causing a substantial inward drain!

While these models exhibit that the different parts or frameworks in the body need distinctive pH levels, we don't have to stress over that.

Our concern is primary, and it's this. We are essential to acidic, generally speaking. In case you're keen on getting familiar with pH, you can discover massive amounts of data on the web by basically searching the term.

The most significant thing to know is this. At the point when your body is too acidic over quite a while, it prompts numerous diseases like stoutness, joint pain, bone thickness loss, hypertension, coronary illness, and stroke. The rundown is unending because the body essentially surrenders the fight for imperativeness and goes into endurance mode for as long as it can.

An alkaline diet is unique.

Numerous diets center on similar nourishments that cause you to be overweight or debilitated in any case. They solicit you to eat less from those things, to eat additional time every day, or to join them quickly.

Indecency to these diet's makers, they realize that vast numbers of us would prefer not to roll out the more significant improvements for our health. We like food that is centered on prepared and refined nourishments, our meat, our sugar, alcohol, and such. The diet makers are attempting to assist us with rolling out more uncomplicated improvements.

We've become acclimated to eating along these lines, and it's not ALL our deficiency! Insatiable nourishment preparing monsters have a personal stake in keeping us eating along these lines. Benefits are a lot higher in this area of the nourishment business than in the generation of your progressively fundamental nourishments like foods grown from the ground.

In this way, once more, YES, this diet is extraordinary. On the off chance that those different diets worked, you would feel lean, healthy, and crucial. You wouldn't have to peruse this article. You wouldn't require a dietary change.

Here's a fractional rundown of nourishments that you can eat unreservedly in an alkaline diet:

- Fresh foods grown from the ground made juices
- Fresh veggies and juices
- Cooked veggies
- Some vegetables and soy
- Lean proteins and a few eggs
- Certain grains
- Healthy fats and nuts

You can expend constrained amounts of these nourishments and refreshments:

- Dairy
- Many normal grains
- Refined nourishments and sugars
- Alcohol and caffeine

What's it like to be on the alkaline diet, and what results would you be able to anticipate?

Like any adjustment in diet or way of life, you'll experience a modification period, however, because you're consuming the cleanest fuel, which your body pines for, so not at all like many diet plans, you won't ever need to feel hungry. Also, you can eat all you like until you're fulfilled. You likewise won't have to check calories. What's more, you'll appreciate a lot of assortment, so you'll never get exhausted with eating.

Think about an alkaline diet as a sort of 'juice quick' for the body. Just it's not all that outrageous. You're eating supplement thick, effectively absorbable nourishment that your body wants. When you give every one of the cells of the body that it so frantically needs, your craving leaves. Also, there's no compelling reason to stress over exhausting veggies since there are vast amounts of delightful recipes found on the web and in books.

With all the diet designs out there, for what reason would it be advisable for you to consider an elective arrangement like the alkaline diet?

When pursued appropriately, you can hope to liquefy the fat away more effectively than with conventional plans. Numerous tributes exist where individuals report shedding more than two pounds every week. (Furthermore, that much weight wouldn't be intelligent in most diet programs.) Plus, your skin will turn out to be increasingly supple once more, your energy will increment, and you'll feel more youthful.

Furthermore, the alkaline diet does two significant things that conventional diets don't.

1. It gives better sustenance than your body's cells.

2. It detoxifies typically and cleanses the cells, as well.

These two certainties are behind the motivation behind why an alkaline diet works so rapidly and securely.

One last note, while thinking about an alkaline diet. Since it tends to be unique about how you might be accustomed to eating, you may think about whether you can come back to your previous dietary patterns. The legit answer is that it's keen to proceed with the same number of the standards as you can once you have lost all your weight. Be that as it may, it shouldn't be win big or bust. Anything you do to receive a healthier diet will significantly expand your odds of keeping the weight off for good. When you pursue an alkaline diet for a month or two, you can decide the amount of it you need to embrace as a significant aspect of your long-haul healthy way of life.

Utilizing an Alkaline Diet for Weight Loss

Numerous individuals endeavor prevailing fashion diets or those which guarantee snappy outcomes trying to get in shape. These diets may create brings about the present moment, yet after some time, this can be an exceptionally unhealthy approach to get thinner. Also, numerous individuals recover the weight when they go off their exacting diet. At the point when an acid diet is utilized for weight loss and control, it is all the more a way of life change. The outcomes may not occur without any forethought. However, the weight won't be recovered. An alkaline diet is wealthy in nourishments, which are generally low in calories, for example, most vegetables and natural products. A significant number of the nourishments that are high in fat and calories are likewise acidifying, so when these nourishments are expelled from the diet, a characteristic and healthy weight loss will happen. These nourishments incorporate red meat, greasy food sources, and high-fat dairy items, for example, whole milk and cheddar, sugar, pop, and liquor. When you quit eating these nourishments, your body will be a lot healthier, less acid, and you'll additionally get more fit all the while. Since the diet is healthy, you can stay with it long haul. Numerous individuals who start an alkaline diet exclusively to get in shape find countless different advantages. An expanded energy level, protection from an ailment, and a general improvement in health and prosperity are among the numerous benefits you can understand on an alkaline diet.

Numerous individuals find that it is simpler to begin an alkaline diet by rolling out little improvements. Start by gradually decreasing the measure of meat, sugar, and fat in your diet, while including crisp organic products, vegetables, healthy fats, for example, olive oil, almonds, soy items, and normal sugars, for instance, Stevia. You'll discover after some time, your preferences will change, and you'll begin to lean toward this sort of diet.

How Your Body Handles Acid

Anyway, for what reason would anyone care about being on an alkaline diet in any case? Well, the explanation is necessary. As a populace, we are tossing our bodies out of equalization by ingesting poisons, for example, pop and creature proteins in mass amounts. Subsequently, acid is developed in such enormous quantities that the body goes into endurance mode. While acid would ordinarily be handled and expelled by the liver and kidneys, when a lot of it exists, the body stores it in fat to save the health of your organs. The outcome is an unequal measure of acid and dehydration in the body. The body's homeostasis exists at a pH estimation of 7.3. Standard (unbiased) water has a pH of 7.0.

The capacity to ionizer water and devour an alkaline diet has incredible advantages for your health.

However, for what reason is an alkaline extraordinary for weight loss? A horde of advantages has been ascribed to keeping up your body's normal ph. Turning around the impacts of continuous diseases, for example, diabetes, acid reflux, angina, headaches, and joint inflammation, are a couple of the significant advantages. Liberating people with diabetes from their insulin crazed appetite fits has brought about a lot of weight loss. However, you'll see that even typical individuals have seen incredible weight loss because of an alkaline diet. At the point when the body is liberated of its harmful express, your digestion can work all the more productively. Fat and proteins are scorched and put away appropriately. Likewise, individuals have seen the advantages of expanded energy and sex drive, enabling them to be increasingly dynamic and gainful.

Improving Your Alkaline Diet for Weight Loss

If you are endeavoring to utilize an alkaline diet for weight loss, it is significant you realize how to adopt the fair strategy. In the fact that you use alkaline water and alkaline nourishments related to a healthy way of life, you will get the "wonder" weight loss that everybody is raving about. When you start drinking the alkaline water all the time, you can move from drinking water with pH 9.0 to pH 9.5 (for grown-ups). Expending a good measure of this high pH water is ensured to help the body in coming back to acid-alkaline congruity. Additionally, you should utilize the high pH water while getting ready nourishments like soup and stews, to adjust the acidifying creature proteins or other acidic parts of the nourishment.

In the above, you have perceived how you can utilize an alkaline diet for weight loss, yet there is significantly more to be scholarly. To guarantee that you are going to lose weight, it is significant you find out about alkaline nourishments. The absolute most acid-filled nourishments would be the ones you wouldn't dare hoping anymore. Numerous dairy items, for instance, are exceptionally high in acid substance.

Alkaline Diet for Health and Weight Loss

There are a ton of insane diets available that guarantee to assist you with shedding pounds. Shockingly, on the off chance that you take a gander at the healthy benefit of a portion of these diets, they are regularly seriously deficient. If you have to get thinner, you ought to do it while eating food that is useful for your body, with the goal that you will get healthier rather than merely more slender. An alkaline diet is a healthy way to deal with weight loss that will keep you stimulated, healthy, and inspired to drop the pounds.

An alkaline diet is not the same as different diets since it centers mostly around the impact that nourishments have on the acidity or the alkalinity of the body. At the point when nourishments are processed and used by the body, they produce what is usually alluded to as an "alkaline debris" or "acid debris." The first pH of the nourishment doesn't factor into this decisive impact inside the body. The absolute most acidic nourishments, for example, organic citrus products, really produce an alkaline effect when eaten. At the point when increasingly alkaline nourishments are eaten instead of acid nourishments, the pH of the body can be acclimated to an ideal degree of roughly 7.3. While this isn't incredibly alkaline, it is sufficient to receive numerous healthful rewards.

Alkaline Diet - How Does It Help?

The alkaline diet, otherwise called Alkaline Acid Diet, is diet-dependent on the utilization of nourishment. For example, natural products, vegetables, roots, nuts, and vegetables, however, maintain a strategic distance from dairy, meat, grains, and salts. As of late, this diet has picked up fame among diet and nourishment experts and creators. It is still in banter on the productivity of the alkaline diet because there is no solid proof that the alkaline diet can decrease certain diseases.

As previously mentioned, organic products, vegetables, roots, nuts, and vegetables are a piece of an alkaline diet. This is because this nourishment discharged alkaline in the wake of being processed, assimilated, and used. Then again, dairy, meat, grains, and salts produce acid after the procedures. Nourishment is classified as acid-delivering or alkaline-creating dependent on their pH (intensity of Hydrogen) values, where pH 0 - 6 is acidic, pH 8 - 14 is alkaline, and pH 7 is nonpartisan (water). Consequently, the alkaline diet alludes to the menu of having a more significant amount of alkaline-delivering nourishment.

Alkaline Diet

Our blood has a pH somewhere in the range of 7.35 and 7.45, which is marginally alkaline. The alkaline diet depends on this pH level of our blood, and any food that is high in acid-delivering nourishment will disorganize the equalization. At the point when the body attempts to rejuvenate the harmony of pH in the blood, the acidity of the food will add to the loss of crucial minerals, for example, potassium, magnesium, calcium, and sodium. The irregularity will make individuals vulnerable to sickness.

Sadly, Western diets are progressively acid-delivering, and they expend minimal new foods grown from the ground. Because of the approach of the alkaline diet, the standard of the Western diet has changed impressively. Some diet and nourishment professionals accept that acid-delivering diet may cause some constant ailment and following manifestations, for example,

- Migraine
- Lazy
- Visit influenza and cold, and overabundance mucous generation
- Tension, apprehension
- Polycystic ovaries, ovarian sores, considerate bosom growths

Albeit some accept the above conditions are the consequence of acid-delivering diet and utilization of products of the soil is valuable to health, a few specialists believe that acid-creating diet doesn't cause persistent disease. Other than that, there are proofs demonstrated that alkaline foods forestall the development of calcium kidney stones, osteoporosis, and age-related muscle squandering.

Albeit an alkaline diet is liked, it isn't prescribed to have an extreme diet (eat all alkaline-delivering nourishment). It is healthier to take a stab at a reasonable center ground of the two kinds of food. Simply make sure to observe the pointers above and counsel a specialist/specialist before you need to attempt another diet.

Step by step instructions to lose weight with an alkaline diet and alkaline foods

Those battling with abundance weight see many commercials of thousands of weight loss items. However, a large portion of these individuals never knows WHY they are overweight in any case. Numerous individuals like to have more energy for the day, yet the tidbits and stimulated drinks that many expend are exceptionally acid shaping.

By making acidity in blood, tissue, and body cells, these ordinary tidbits (just as cheap food, handled nourishment, desserts, all yeast containing items, and so forth.) may meddle with healthy energy creation and frequently bring about ensuing weight gain. The purpose behind that is the body's reaction to overabundance acidity: it stores acid squanders in fat cells to keep them from essential organs.

The over-acidification/acidosis of our body cells is the purpose behind numerous diseases, will hinder cell exercises and works, and is the thing that prompts overweight: to shield itself from conceivably genuine harm, the body makes new fat cells to store the additional acid. Be that as it may, when the acidic condition is wiped out, the fat inside the body is never again required, and dissolves away.

The body's inside condition is somewhat alkaline, which is the reason it requests a diet that is likewise marginally alkaline. The body's whole metabolic procedure relies upon a chemical situation. Our inner framework lives and bites the dust at the cell level, every one of the billions of cells that make up the human body is somewhat alkaline and must keep up alkalinity to work and stay healthy and alive.

Alkaline Food will cause nourishment desires to die down usually because the acidity inside the inner condition is killed through the alkaline framing components. When the internal landscape is alkalized with alkaline water and essential nourishment as indicated by an alkaline diet (=weight loss diet), the body is allowed to discharge the acid waste and copies of fat. Along these lines, your pH level will likewise be adjusted, and each organ capacities better, supporting healthy digestion and making weight control a lot simpler.

What are the Results of the Alkaline Diet?

When an alkaline diet is begun, the vast majority find that their pH usually turns out to be increasingly caustic. One gets the opportunity to perceive how particular kinds of dinners make an exceptionally acidic condition and figure out how to change their dietary patterns to more readily bolster weight control. At the point when pH balance is accomplished through essential nourishment and basic nutritional habits, the body drops typically to its healthy weight, nourishment longings will decrease, glucose levels are adjusted, and energy levels will increment monstrously.

So, anyone prepared to seek after the way of better health, weight loss, and more energy ought to consider the upsides of the alkaline diet for accomplishing an ideal pH balance in the body. It is perfect for anybody anxious to fabricate an establishment for good health - presently and for the years to come. Equalization pH-Diet.com illuminates individuals about the over-acidification of the body because of quick-paced and unhealthy ways of life, which is the purpose behind numerous diseases and weight gain.

Alkaline Diet Can Save Your Life

The theory behind the alkaline diet is that because the pH of our body is somewhat salty, with an ordinary scope of 7.36 to 7.44, our food ought to mirror this and be marginally soluble. An unequal diet high in acidic nourishments like creature protein, caffeine, sugar, and handled nourishments will, in general, upset this equalization. It can drain the collection of alkaline minerals, for example, sodium, potassium, magnesium, and calcium, making individuals helpless against interminable and degenerative diseases.

Our inner concoction balance is fundamentally constrained by our lungs, kidneys, digestive organs, and skin. For fundamental capacities to happen, our body must keep up an appropriate pH. The proportion of the acidity or alkalinity of a substance is called pH. Sufficient alkaline stores are required for the ideal alteration of pH. The body needs oxygen, water, and acid-buffering minerals to achieve the pH-buffering while rapidly evacuating waste items.

The over-acidification of the body is the fundamental reason for all diseases. Soft drink is presumably the most acidic nourishment individuals expend at a pH of 2.5. Soft drink is multiple times more acidic than nonpartisan water and takes 32 glasses of impartial water to adjust a glass of pop. Alkaline nourishment and water ought to be devoured, to give supplements the body needs to kill acids and poisons from the blood, lymph, and tissues, and simultaneously, reinforces the safe and organ frameworks.

Most vegetables and organic products contain a higher measure of essential shaping components than different nourishments. The more noteworthy the ratio of green nourishments devoured in the diet, the more prominent the health benefits are accomplished. These plant nourishments are purifying and alkalizing to the body, while the refined and handled nourishments can increment unhealthy degrees of acidity and poisons. Be that as it may, know that an excess of alkaline can likewise hurt you. You should have the best possible information on adjusting alkaline and acidic nourishments in your diet. After ingestion, alkaline nourishment and water are very quickly killed by hydrochloric acid present in the stomach. The harmony among alkaline and acidic nourishments must be kept up all together for your organs to perform well.

A healthy and adjusted diet is more alkaline than acid. Given your blood classification, the menu ought to be comprised of 60 to 80% alkaline nourishments and 20 to 40% acidic food sources. Typically, the A and AB blood classifications require the most alkaline diet, while the O and B blood classifications require creature items increasingly in their diet. In any case, remember, in case you're in torment, you're acidic. Progressing to an alkaline diet requires a move in one's mentality about nourishment. It is useful to investigate new tastes and surfaces while rolling out little improvements and improving old propensities.

Ideal Health Through the Alkaline Diet

The alkaline diet, acid alkaline diet, or alkaline acid diet is a kind of food that spotlights on the utilization of crisp vegetables, new organic products, root crops, tubers, vegetables, nuts, and every so often fish. By enjoying this sort of diet, it's accepted by the diet's specialists that we forestall the risks of acidity.

Returning to the Past

Ancient man expended a diet that bears little likenesses from the foods we devour today. Their diets are comprised of wild vegetation and meat from prey. After the revelation of horticulture around 10,000 years prior, this diet changed.

After stone devices were created, grains turned into a reasonable nourishment source. When filtering and moving gadgets were designed, refined grains were presented. Dairy items were found when creatures were trained, thus did the measure of promptly accessible meat sources. Salt for enhancing was additionally found. During the mechanical upset, sugar as a sugar turned out to be mainstream.

The Reality

Nourishment, when processed, is either acidic or alkaline. There ought to be a harmony between the two. Sadly, because of the headways of horticulture and how we process nourishment and progress, we expend progressively acidic nourishment types contrasted with alkaline. The procedure that should keep us all around encouraged is, unfortunately, the reason for our very own end.

Blood coursing through our veins ought to be kept up somewhat alkaline. The pH levels in blood ought to in a perfect world be at 7.35 to 7.45. Professionals of the alkaline diet resolutely express that the type of food you eat will affect your general health. This implies acidic nourishment makes ready for diseases like diabetes and cancer, and alkaline framing nourishment makes available to consummate health.

Chapter 6: How to Know That Your Detox Diet is Working

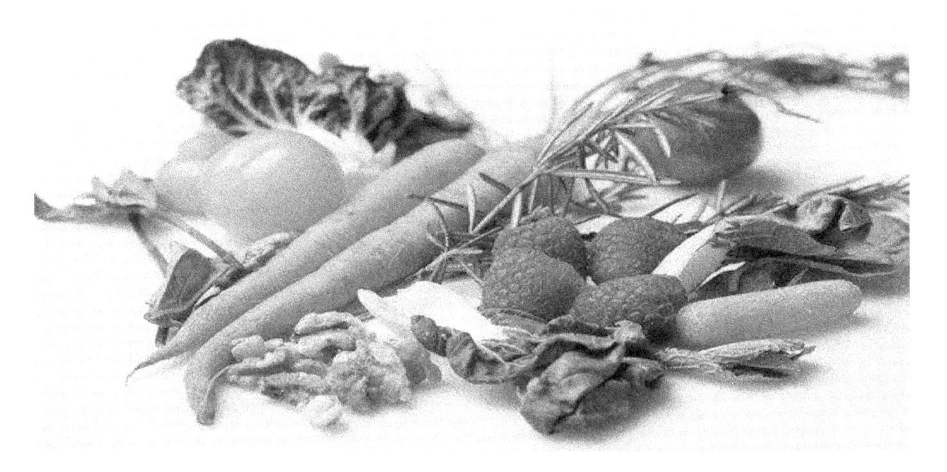

What Is Cleansing or Detoxification?

Cleansing or detoxification is an alternative medication used in getting rid of all the acidic and toxins content (mucus) that have accumulated in the body which have made the body system to be vulnerable to disease. Until we stop eating; preserved/canned food, our body will be filled with toxins that have either short- or long-term effects on the human's health. However, the way to a healthy, happy, and sick-free lifestyle, is to cleanse or detoxify the body system of all the toxic which makes the body vulnerable to disease.

How Do I Undergo A Cleanse?

When talking about cleansing, most doctors will only talk about the cleansing of the colon but Dr. Sebi, disagree with their opinion and state that, to do a cleanse, you will need to do an intra-cellular cleansing. That is, cleansing of each cell from the body system. However, to do an intra-cellular cleansing, you will need to cleanse the following:

i. Colon.

ii. Lymphatic gland

iii. Skin

iv. Kidney v. Liver and

vi. Gallbladder

What Are the Various Types of Cleansing?

Although there are various types of detoxification, I am going to center on fasting which is the one approved by late Dr. Sebi.

Under the fasting method of detoxification, there are various types of fasting which include:

Dry fasting

Under this type of fasting, you will abstain from food, water, juice, anything eatable or drinkable.

Liquid fasting

under this type of fasting, you are to abstain from anything solid and consume only liquid-like; juice and any other liquid stuff without alcohol.

Water fasting

under this type of fasting, you are to abstain from anything solid, juice, smoothies, etc. and consume only water.

Fruit fasting

under this type of fasting, you are to avoid anything solid but survive mainly on fruit.

Raw food fasting

under this type of fasting, you are to abstain completely from cooked food and survive mainly on veggies and fruit.

Smoothie fasting

smoothie fasting is just like the fruit fasting, the only difference is the fact that under smoothie fasting, the fruit will be blended, and you will also consume blended veggies.

Bear in mind that, Dr. Sebi approved 12 days fast with alkaline herbs, sea moss, spring water, and green smoothies which must be made with fruit that are in Dr. Sebi's nutritional guide list.

Body detox

Since Dr. Sebi's diet contains alkaline-based foods, some of them assist in reducing the inflammations in the kidney. Other meals such as the marshmallows are diuretic; hence, they boost the amount of urine your body produces. The body then flushes out the particles from the kidney. Diets containing parsley helps in preventing kidney stones. As a result, the kidney's functions are done with ease.

Potassium-rich foods for liver health

- Raisins
- Almond
- Dulse
- Prunes
- Kelp
- Banana

Juices and raw vegetables for liver health

- Plum tomatoes
- Asparagus
- Okra
- Cabbage
- Rosemary
- Amaranth greens
- Dandelion greens

- Fennel

Fruit juices are excellent nutrients for liver function

- Ginger juice
- Lemon juice
- Fresh prune juice
- Apple juice

The importance of water

- Water assists in hydrating the body.
- The function of natural foods
- Asparagus invigorates the capacity of the liver.
- Ginger shields the liver as it contains eight exacerbates.
- Prune juice flushes each debasement from the liver Apples make the liver productive in its procedure's Dandelion washes down the liver
- Rosemary helps restores a feeble liver

Herbs for liver health

- Lobelia
- Parsley
- Yellow dock
- Dandelion

- Bayberry

Before You Begin

There are many different types of cleanses, from fasting to whole foods, but they all aim to accomplish the same thing, and that is to get rid of inflammatory substances and toxicity. Then they provide your body with pure forms of nutrients. The goal of a cleanse is to heal and restore your body to its optimal health and give its powerful detoxification systems to work without the blockages that are normally there.

The occasional detox is great for the body, but you should never just jump straight into a detox. Getting your body ready for the detox is just as important as the actual detox. If you already follow a very healthy and clean diet, then you won't have as much to do to get ready. But if you are like most people and follow a standard American diet, then you will have some work to do.

Cleanse and detox are words that tend to be used interchangeably, but they aren't quite the same thing. A cleanse is something that you do that will cause detoxification. Your body detoxes naturally as soon as your food has been digesting. This is where it will remove toxic and foreign materials. Unfortunately, the regular lifestyle and diets of most people cause them to accumulate more toxins than the body is able to purge. Because of this, we need to, on occasion, do a cleanse or fast where we consciously reduce the number of toxins that we are consuming so that the body is forced into a natural detoxifying state.

A cleanse could be a complete abstinence from food or toxic activities, and you only consume water. This type of fast might be helpful, but it's pretty hard to keep up. The Dr. Sebi detox won't require you to stop eating altogether, but if you want to try that type of cleanse, feel free to because it can do amazing things to your body.

Starting just a few days before you plan on beginning your detox, you will want to start changing how you eat. You will need to eat simple, light foods like salads, soups, or veggies. You will want to focus on raw veggies and leafy greens. This is especially true if you haven't been much of a clean eater. You need to give your body a chance to get ready for the cleanse. Take little steps by slowly cutting out processed and sugar foods, and start to increase your intake of fresh foods and grains.

Taking these small steps will increase your body's alkalinity to help it get ready for the deeper cleanse of your detox. During the detox, your body is going to end up releasing toxins that are stored in your tissues. These toxins may enter your bloodstream and can end up causing trouble sleeping, mood swings, body odor, bad breath, aches, and pains, or rashes. By preparing for your detox, you can minimize your chances of developing these side effects.

To help you out, we will go over some tips on getting your body ready for your detox.

Begin Your Day Right

You should start adding in a glass of warm lime water to your daily routine. This helps to jump-start your digestion and boost your metabolism. Lime juice is very alkalizing to your body, rich in vitamin C, and helps to cleanse your liver, which are all very important parts of detoxification.

Switch Up Your Drinks

You will want to start drinking more spring water during the day and start adding in some cleansing herbal teas, such as burdock, dandelion root, or nettle tea. This is also the best time to switch from regular tap water to spring water. You have to drink spring water while on Dr. Sebi's detox.

If you drink alcohol or coffee, you need to start cutting back on your consumption of them. You won't be able to have them on the detox. To let go of coffee, a good alternative is herbal or green tea. While green tea does contain caffeine, it is full of antioxidants, which will help your detoxification. Sodas and energy drinks should also be eliminated.

Water will play a very big part in your life, so beginning your day with two glasses of water is helpful in getting ready for your detox. If you choose to do the hot lime water, that counts towards a glass.

Keep Things Simple

Starting to change your meals to something that is very simple and easy to make. You should opt for dishes that are heavy in natural fruits and vegetables and start weaning yourself off of meats if you are a meat-eater. Include a lot of foods that are rich in chlorophyll because these aid in detoxification.

This can also include drinking veggie soups and broths. If you find it hard to eat enough vegetables, you can get your veggie intake through smoothies or juice. An easy way to add more fruits and veggies into your current diet is by adding a piece of organic fresh fruit to your breakfast each morning. You can also turn to fresh fruits as your mid-afternoon snack instead of heading to the vending machine. When picking out your fruits and veggies, go with organic, seasonal, and local produce when you can so that you avoid pesticides.

Reduce Your Animal Product Intake

You are going to have to cut out animal products completely on Dr. Sebi's fast, so leading up to it, you should start weaning yourself off of them. The first place to start is to stop eating processed and red meats. This includes things like cured meats and sausages. Choosing leaner meats and fish is a better choice during this time. When picking fish, stay away from fish that are high in mercury, like mackerel and tuna. Fish like salmon, scallops, anchovies, and shrimp are better options.

Check Your Oils

A lot of people will cook with vegetable or canola oil because the health industry tells you they are better because they are lower in fat, but they aren't. You need to start using olive oil, avocado oil, coconut oil, and grapeseed oil. Coconut and olive oils should not be cooked and should only be used raw. You can also use these oils along with some lime juice and herbs to create your own salad dressings.

Up Your Grain Intake

Right now, you don't have to worry about eating Dr. Sebi approved grains. All you need to worry about is increasing how much whole grains you eat. Start eating more brown rice or spelt, and also start eating more pseudo-grains like quinoa. You need to start reducing how many refined foods like pasta and bread you consume, and that includes whole-grain bread or pasta. Do your best to avoid wheat wherever you are able to.

Get Rid of Refined Sugar

You have to start reading nutrition levels to make sure that foods aren't hiding sugars. Before the detox, you can pick healthier sugar alternatives in moderation. Maple syrup, raw honey, rapadura sugar, coconut blossom syrup, coconut sugar, or agave nectar are great alternatives. Once the detox starts, you will only be able to have agave nectar.

Get Rid of Table Salt

Table salt does not provide you with any nutrients. Your body also has a very hard time metabolizing table salt. While you are checking nutrition labels for sugars, check and make sure they aren't hiding any table salts. The majority of processed foods will have large amounts of chemically processed salts. You should use sea salt as your salt source. It is full of minerals and they are able to help get rid of heavy metals within your body.

Cut Out Unhealthy Foods

Leading up to the detox, you should slowly start cutting out unhealthy foods that you like to eat. This includes things like store-bought cookies or muffins, chips, and fried foods. Choose, instead, to snack on homemade dried fruit, seeds, and unsalted nuts. Before the detox, feel free to try some raw chocolate to help you with your chocolate fix.

Get Your Mind Ready

But what should we do about the mind? There is a lot of evidence that has found that our mental state, from stressed to relaxed and all that is in between, has a large impact on our wellbeing and health. While you can do a cleanse for a week without changing anything else about your day, and you may feel pretty good after, but, when you add mindfulness into your cleanse, you will uncover some amazing opportunities to move your focus inwards to create as much space in your emotional body and mind as you can in the physical body.

You could possibly be at a time of transition and you're looking for a fresh start to push yourself into the next phase. You could be holding onto something, such as a loss, fear, resentment, or unhealthy relationship, that you want to get rid of. Maybe most of your day is spent focusing on and caring for other people and feel like you need to do something for yourself. A lot of use resist turning in and may even fear it. You could have an inner voice asking you to stop distracting yourself in order to listen to your intuition.

In order to get the most from your cleanse, it is a good idea to like what you want to get rid of other than the junk in your diet, and why you are drawn to this cleanse.

Relax and Meditate

Getting ready for the cleanse doesn't just mean getting your belly ready for the change in foods, but it also means making sure your mind is ready for the change. Relaxation and mediation are a big part of detoxing because they can help you to reduce or eliminate your stress. Stress is the number one cause of so many unhealthy habits, such as snacking on junk food or overeating. If you simply set aside some time each day to simply sit and be still, it will help to quiet your mind. This will help you to remain focused on what your goals are.

Start Journaling

It's also a good idea to start keeping a detox journal. While you are getting ready for your detox, you can take the time to write out the guidelines for it, or simply write out what you hope it will do for you. In it, you should also make sure you schedule rest time. Your body will be doing a lot of work, and it's common to start feeling tired. Making sure you have rest time set aside will help to combat any fatigue you may experience. While detoxing, you can expel mental toxins by writing in the journal. You can write anything you want so that you mentally cleanse yourself. Let the words flow and don't worry if it makes sense, is grammatically correct, or what have you. Simply writing things out on paper is very therapeutic.

Clear Your Space

While this might not seem important, but before you start cleaning your insides, you should also clean your outside. It has been proven that the health of the mind is greatly impacted by your surroundings and all of the environmental toxins lurking in your space. Take the time to vacuum the floor, give your sheets a change, and use an air filter. You should also create your own sanctuary that you can use during your cleanse. This could be an entire room in your house, if you have a spare one, or it could simply be a comfy chair placed next to a window. Wherever you place your sanctuary, remove all of the clutter and place a vase of some of your favorite flowers or simply a photo that makes you happy. You can also choose something that calms or inspires you.

Let Your Family and Friends Know

You are getting ready to embark on something that is likely going to be very different from your everyday life. That means anybody you socialize with on a regular basis is probably going to notice something. Those that you live with will definitely notice something. To make sure that you are successful at your cleanse you will want to let your inner circle know what you are doing. Make sure that you get everybody on the same page so that they will know why you can't do certain things or go out to certain places during your weeklong cleanse. Your closest friends and family tend to be your biggest cheerleaders, so they may just be the person you turn to when you feel like giving up.

That being said, don't be surprised if one of them questions you about your choice to cleanse. If this happens, simply explain to them why you want to do this. If that's not good enough for them, don't try to change their mind. You don't have to have their approval to do this. You are doing this only for you, and not for them. If you have to keep your distance from them during the cleanse, then do so. Do what is best for you.

Change Up Your Inner Dialogue

You know all of the negativity that tends to be swarming around in your head? You know that defeatist inner monologue that everybody tends to slip into from time to time? Now, is all of that serving you at all? When you start telling yourself that you aren't good enough, smart enough, skinny enough, and so, does it help you reach your goals? It is now time for you to change that inner dialogue. What though patterns will you be able to let go of as you are cleansing? To help you out, try writing down the negative things that you have told yourself. Underneath that negative thought, in bigger letters, change that negative sentence into a positive one. Things like "I can do anything I set my mind to," "I am worthy," or "I am beautiful the way I am" are all great choices. You should also think about making this your mantra for your cleanse. You should say this out loud each and every day. At first, you might not believe the words coming out of your mouth, but after a while, you will start to believe it.

Pick a Good Time

While there likely is no perfect time to do a detox, it's a good idea to look at your calendar to see when you have free time. If you do, by chance, of a week of vacation built up at work and haven't made any other plans that might be a good option that way you don't have to worry about work. It's also a good idea to make sure that you detox won't occur during any major life events, holidays, important projects at work, or vacations. You definitely don't want to have a marathon run scheduled during the time you plan on doing your detox. It is just for a week, so it shouldn't be too hard to find at least one week where you don't have a lot going on.

Think About a Digital Detox

This isn't something that you have to do, but it might be a good option if you are able to. Try to go digital-free for at least one whole day during your cleanse. The majority of people carry incredible power around with us in the form of tiny computers in your pocket. Remember, this cleanse that you have planned is time that you have set aside for yourself in order to remove junk from your life and replenish your system with healthy things.

This is true for your mind just as much as it is for your entire body. When you are going to the gym or heading out somewhere, leave your phone at home. Switch off your social media notifications. Choose one or two hours during the day to go through your emails or create an away message to let people know that you will get back to them tomorrow. Now that you have carved out some undistracted time, do something fun or healthy, like reading a book, write a letter, take a walk, or work on that project you have been meaning to for months. Whatever you want to do, that doesn't have to do with the digital world, do it.

Lean into Your Breath

When you start to experience the emotional or physical side effects of the cleanse, take a few minutes to simply breathe so that you can connect with your body. This will help to slow your heart rate, help you to deal with imagined or real hunger, push through your erratic energy or mood swing, and then move the focus on your mind back into focus.

To do this, all you need to do is either stand or sit still and let your eyes close gently or leave them open if you need to. Then take ten deep breaths in through your nose and release them out your mouth. As you inhale, picture it as a cleansing energy and view your exhalation as a release of negativity. This can easily be done anywhere, like sitting in traffic or at the grocery store. Simply moving your attention to the movement of your breath will help to bring you into the present moment.

Find a Cleanse Buddy

This might not be possible but see if you can create some support for yourself and find somebody to do the cleanse with you. While a week may not sound that long, there may be times when it feels longer because it is so different from what your body is used to. Ask some of your friends and family, or even see there is a Facebook group of people who would like to do the cleanse with you.

You will add extra incentive to reach your goal when you have another person holding you accountable, or if there some fun competition added in. You don't have to be in the state, or even the same country to do this. As long as two or more of you can stay in contact with each other, that's all that matters. Check in every few hours, or at least send a picture to one another of what you are eating.

Get Your Fridge Ready

Once you feel that you have sufficiently gotten your body and mind ready for your cleanse, you need to move onto your refrigerator. To ensure success, you will want to make sure that you have gotten rid of all of the temptations that you can by going through your fridge and cabinets.

The first thing you should do is make sure that your fridge is full of Dr. Sebi approved vegetables and fruits so that you will have what you need on hand for your fast. It's a good idea to have the fruits and veggies prepared in a way that makes it easy to just grab and use them. You can also go ahead and mix up your juices and smoothies that you will need for the week as well. You could also just have what you need for your juices and smoothies diced and in containers where all you have to do it throw it in the blender and go. When you have all of your food ready to go, it will save you some time in preparing your meals. It also means, if you start feeling hungry before you are supposed to eat next, you will have a quick snack that you can grab. This will lower the odds of you grabbing something not so healthy.

If you live with other people who won't be doing this cleanse with you, then you may not be able to throw out all of the bad foods. If they have snacks that don't have to be refrigerated, ask them to put them up somewhere so that you can't see them and don't know where they are. It may also be a good idea to keep your food separate from theirs in the fridge. This just ensures the things you need for the week don't get used up by accident.

You can prep any salads you may need for the week by fixing them in a mason jar. Make sure that the dressing is placed on the bottom and everything is stacked on top. Also, have a gallon of spring water drawn up at the end of each day ready for the next day. It is also a good idea to have a glass of water with you during the day. This can help with the hunger you might experience.

Be Easy on Yourself

We are all just human. We aren't perfect and messing up happens even if we have planned as much as we can. If you find that you end up giving into temptation and mess up a bit, don't simply throw in the towel and give up. The cup of coffee or that piece of chocolate doesn't mean you're a failure and does not mean you should stop your cleanse. A slip up may slow down your progress, but it does not bring it to a stop.

You are doing this cleanse for you and nobody else. If you slip, realize what happened, and then get back on track for your next meal. You may even notice that eating "off cleanse" makes you feel crappy. You may feel like your energy slumped, you develop of headache, or you may feel bloated. When this happens, simply recommit. Remind yourself of what your goal is and then remember that the next meal you have is another chance to make a different choice.

Before you start the cleanse take a picture of yourself from angles, measure your chest, waist, hips, upper arm, and thighs, and weight yourself. Also, write down how you have been feeling before the detox, such as tired, bloated, sluggish, and so on. During the detox, and this plays into your journaling, you can keep track of how you feel each day. Try to avoid re-measuring or weighing yourself during the detox. Then the morning of the first day off of the cleanse, so the eighth day, take new pictures, measurements, and weight. Then jot down how you are feeling. Do you have more energy? Do you feel motivated to eat healthier? Did you enjoy your experience? And so on.

The most effective method to detox your body naturally

Figuring out how to detox your body [can have a significant effect on your health and prosperity. We are assaulted with poisons at consistently expanding rates from the air we inhale and the nourishment we eat. So, following a healthy detox diet program at regular intervals is turning out to be progressively significant consistently. Begin today.

Herbs That Detox the Body Quickly

Everybody realizes that it is so critical to detox your body usually, supposing that you don't then poisons develop and this can have transient consequences for you, for example, tiredness, laziness, and absence of energy and even some long haul impacts, for example, expanded danger of specific disease.

There is a lot of costly detox medicines accessible. Yet, little to individuals realize that the absolute best detox specialists are exceptionally modest and can be found in your ordinary market or store. These herbs that detox the body are beneficial for your body and won't just assist it with detoxing; however, will likewise give you better by and abundant health, expanded energy, and a more grounded safe framework.

All in all, what are the best herbs that detox the body?

Burdock

This is incredible for detoxing; burdock attaches truly help to decrease the development of substantial metals in your framework, which won't just cleanse your arrangement of these undesirable poisons yet will diminish the danger of safe framework issues later on.

Nettles

Sounds frightful, I know, yet Nettles have some extremely extraordinary detox properties. One of the principle preferences of this herb is that it will cleanse your urinary framework and will counteract any future issues happening.

Milk Thistle

Of the considerable number of herbs that detox the body, this one is most likely one of only a handful, not many that truly helps protein combination in your liver. It will fortify this procedure and make it work considerably more productively.

Dandelion

Dandelion pulls are incredible cleansers for your nerve bladder and liver and will keep them healthy and clean.

Psyllium Seeds

These seeds advance healthy solid discharges and guarantee that everything stays working effectively. This is one of only a handful of scarcely any herbs that detox the body that demonstrations like a kind of wipe and truly helps to wipe up undesirable poisons before being expelled from the body.

For what reason do we need to detox the body?

Detoxification is turning out to be increasingly more significant as time passes by, there are 300,000 new poisons/polluting influences compromising the body every year. That is 6,000 per week that are being added to the Chemical Society's Chemical Abstract. These poisons, some undeniable and some covered up, are making our bodies acidic. In an acidic domain, the disease develops and spreads, anything from the regular cold to cancer contingent upon how poisonous/acidic your body is.

These poisons are surrounding us, it is anything but an instance of escaping from them which would be virtually unimaginable except if you secured yourself a cleaned hatchery yet monitoring them and decreasing the sum you open your body to these harming synthetic concoctions. Alright, so were all mindful of certain poisons, for example, liquor, smoking, drugs, carbon dioxide noticeable all around we breathe, and so forth. However, the dangerous ones are the ones we didn't even know we were expending, i.e.

Medicine

the solution and non-physician endorsed drugs are risky, and inside the body become an exceptionally poisonous acid, making the body progressively acidic; the more acidic you are, the more defenseless against disease you become.

Water

The water we drink contains chlorine.... but chlorine is utilized to kill living beings in our pools; last time I looked, we were a living being? Likewise, ongoing investigations propose to have discovered antidepressants and conception prevention drug in the water we drink.

Skin

Nobody likes to smell, however, in the antiperspirant and antiperspirants we use is a concoction called aluminum cholorohydrate, which is legitimately connected with bosom cancer, to such a degree, that numerous produces have prohibited this from being utilized and gone for the more "characteristic" way!

Diet items

One of the most significant misinterpretations is that "diet" items assist us with getting more fit when everything they do is make us fatter and progressively dangerous. In diet soft drinks, for instance, the ordinary sugar utilized in standard items has been taken out yet lamentably been supplanted with a compound turning out to be increasingly more well-known called Aspartame (there are more than 92 distinctive health indications related to aspartame) which is multiple times better than sugar. At 86 °f, aspartame is separated into another compound formaldehyde. The temperature of the body is 98.6 degrees Fahrenheit! Formaldehyde is utilized as a treating specialist who prevents the body from deteriorating; Formaldehyde can arrive in a glass holder alongside a significant red sign saying DANGER!!

Nourishment

The number of inhabitants on the planet is expanding a seemingly endless amount of time after a year, putting nourishment organizations/ranchers compelled to deliver more nourishment and speedier and with a more drawn out rack life......when was the last time you saw your milkman? We used to get fresh milk delivered each morning; however, now the milk will last as long as seven days. Why? The additives put in our nourishment give it a more extended timeframe of realistic usability because there is such a significant amount of rivalry for our custom added substances are utilized to get you dependent on that specific brand, we as a whole know the motto for Pringles: "When you pop. You can't stop." You will pop if you don't stop! The nourishment we presently expend is of the most awkward things to our health; we can get an entire supper that can be kept for a year and afterward prepared in a short time?? How does that work? Nutritional value, zero! We are eating extraordinary nourishment to what our folks ate and what their people ate. As the nature of food has disintegrated throughout the years, disease has been on the expansion.

Stress

When the body is focused on climate, physical, mental, or enthusiastic, it discharges a hormone called cortisol. Cortisol is a poison to the collection and builds fat stockpiling by expanding your hunger for high fat and high carbohydrate nourishments, and you become a thick putting away machine when focused. Cortisol debilitates your resistant framework by making your body progressively acidic and leaving you increasingly vulnerable to disease.

So, to separate it, the more poisons you take in, the more acidic you become, and the more acidic you are, the almost certain you are to get cancer! Detox intends to dispose of poisons. The body detoxifies typically itself. Still, since of the measure of poisons, the body takes in the liver which is the primary detoxifying organ in the body battles to adapt and only like a shower when it's full, and the tap is as yet running the poisons flood into the body causing acidic/harmful situations. Our body's normal PH levels are 7.34, but since of the measure of poisons, we are presented to our bodies to move into an acidic state regularly. As you most likely are aware, now in an acidic domain, microscopic organisms and disease will develop.

The body's characteristic guard is to clutch any water that you take in to adjust the acid/alkaline levels, causing an additional couple of pounds of water maintenance. The amount of times I've heard individuals state, "On the off chance that I could simply lose two or three pounds." They're most likely clutching 5lbs of water maintenance given the poisons they store in the body.

Recall the poisons we take in are an acid; because we're taking it in limited quantities, it doesn't mean it's not seriously affecting our health. Sadly, when we have been determined to have something is the point at which we begin to respond to it. I generally state be PRO dynamic, not RE dynamic. So how would we do it, we need the most alkaline characteristic enhancements that are accessible to us;

- Stage 1 in our healthy starter packs, we utilize natural herbs like psyllium structures, burdock, dark pecan, cascara, blackthorn, gentian and peony, and others to detox the body and dispose of all the danger that has developed inside you. This will detox your liver, kidneys, colon, and fat stores that store poisons. This will keep going for ten days; you will consider changes to be ahead of schedule as the third or fourth day.

- Stage 2 to be done simultaneously and proceeded after the initial multi-days is to fuse fluid chlorophyll, chlorophyll advances the natural purifying elements of the body, reinforces cells, and freshens up the body, including the bowl. Blend 1 teaspoon (5ml) liquid chlorophyll with water twice every day. Notwithstanding its extraordinary mending properties, chlorophyll is nontoxic and incredible for the entire family to utilize.
- Stage 3, after the underlying ten days of taking acidity out, were going to return in great microorganisms to secure us, and this comes as acidophilus, which is usually found inside the intestinal tract, however, poisons and prescription wipe these out. Each case gives 3.5 billion advantageous microbes to the body. Two containers to be taken twice day by day.

This extremely viable detox can be made significantly progressively feasible whenever pursued by our natural detox diet.

Detoxing benefits

- Increased energy
- Weight loss and increment indigestion
- Clearer skin and improved complexion

- Improved insusceptible framework
- Increased fixation
- Improved absorption
- Strengthens the body's battle against cancer cells and produces healthy cells
- Purify the blood
- Cellulite decrease

Different organs that get detoxed incorporate the kidneys, circulation system, colon, lymphatic framework, thrusts, and skin. Recall detoxing your bodies resembles taking your vehicle for assistance, and how frequently do you do that?

Chapter 7: Dr. Sebi Approved Foods

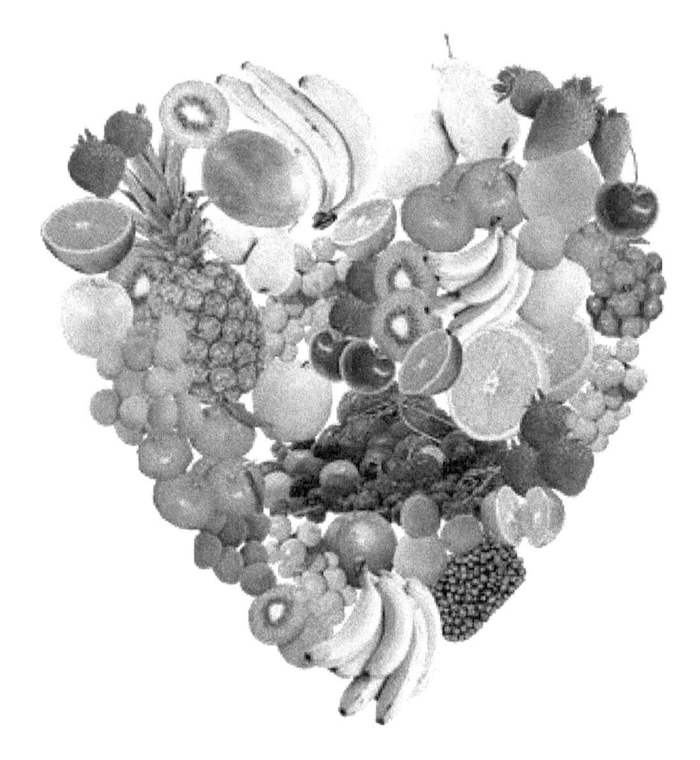

Here is a list of foods permitted by Dr. Sebi's diet for consumption. They are also called the nutritional guide of Dr. Sebi's alkaline diet.

Vegetables that you are allowed to consume

1. Leaves of the amaranth plant

2. Avocado

3. Bell pepper

4. Mexican squash or chayote

5. Cucumbers

6. Dandelion greens

7. Garbanzo beans

8. Cactus leaves and flowers

9. Kale

10. Except for iceberg, all lettuce

11. Except for shitake, all mushrooms

12. Okra

13. Olives

14. Onions

15. Vegetables acquired by the sea, like nori

16. Tomato, only the cherry, and plum kind

17. Greens of turnip

18. Zucchini

19. Water crease

20. Wild arugula

Fruits that you are allowed to consume

1. Apples

2. Bananas

3. Except for cranberries, all berries

4. Cantaloupe

5. Elderberries

6. Cherries

7. Currents

8. Dates

9. Figs

10. Grapes (only seeded are allowed, non-seeded ones are not permitted to be consumed)

11. Mango

12. Melons (only seeded are allowed, non-seeded ones are not permitted to be consumed)

13. Orange, sour ones

14. Papayas

15. Peaches

16. Plums

17. Pears

18. Cactus fruit

19. Tamarinds

20. Soft jelly coconuts

21. Soursop from the Latin or West Indians

22. Raisins (only seeded are allowed, non-seeded ones are not permitted to be consumed)

Tea leaves that you are allowed to consume

1. Burdock
2. Chamomile
3. Elderberry
4. Fennel
5. Ginger
6. Raspberry
7. Tila

Grains that you are allowed to consume

1. Amaranth
2. Fonio
3. Kamut
4. Quinoa
5. Rye
6. Spelt
7. Teff

8. Wild rice

Nuts and seeds that you are allowed to consume

1. Hemp seeds
2. Brazil nuts
3. Walnuts
4. Raw sesame seeds
5. Raw sesame "tahini" seeds

Oils that you are allowed to consume

1. Olive oil (it can only be used as a dressing over dishes, and it is not permitted to be used in cooking)
2. Coconut oil (it can only be used as a dressing over dishes, and it is not permitted to be used in cooking)
3. Hemp seed oil
4. Avocado oil
5. Sesame oil
6. Grapeseed oil

Spices and Condiments that you are allowed to consume

Mild-flavored spices

1. Basil

2. Bay leaf

3. Cloves

4. Thyme

5. Oregano

6. Dill

7. Savory

8. Sweet basil

9. Tarragon

Spicy flavors

1. Achiote

2. African Bird pepper or cayenne pepper

3. Habanero

4. Sage

5. Onion powder

Salty flavors

1. Sea salt (must be pure and not processed at all)

2. Granulated seaweed (can be consumed in powder form)

3. Kelp, nori, or any other seaweed (they can have a sea taste, which might not be very appealing)

Sweet flavors

1. Agave syrup, which is extracted from cactus (must be pure and not processed at all)

2. Date sugar

The entire list of edibles that can be consumed on this diet has been mentioned. Even though it is very restricted, and many fruits and vegetables are banned from the diet, you can still make several versatile dishes to fill your appetite. The focus should be on eating several times throughout the day rather than eating a lot just one time; however, there is no guideline in the diet that tells us when to eat. Be sure to include enough calories from the listed food that fulfills your daily requirements.

Foods to Avoid on the Diet

Foods that are not listed in the nutritional guide are not allowed to be consumed. Some examples of such foods are given below:

1. Any canned product, be it fruits or vegetables, listed in the nutritional guide

2. Seedless fruits like grapes

3. Eggs are not permitted

4. Any type of dairy product is not allowed

5. Fish is not permitted

6. Any type of poultry is not to be eaten

7. Red meat is strictly banned

8. Soy products, which are a replacement for meat, are also banned

9. Processed foods are not allowed

10. Restaurant foods and delivered foods are not to be consumed

11. Hybrid and fortified foods are not permitted

12. Wheat is not permitted

13. White sugar is strictly banned

14. Alcohol is banned

15. Yeast and its products are not allowed

16. Baking powder is not permitted

Some other foods and ingredients have been cut off. You only need to follow the nutritional guide to know what you have to eat.

Every fruit and all the non-starchy vegetables are going to have an alkaline-forming effect on our bodies. This means that potatoes and bananas are more acidic than other fruits and vegetables. Due to this, most berries, non-starchy vegetables, and fruits have to be what you eat the most of. Nature has made it so that bell peppers and leafy greens like kale are extremely alkaline. These are the most nutrient-dense foods that we can eat.

Refined and whole grains will have an acidic effect on our bodies. Legumes are what is called semi-alkaline. All fish, sugar, eggs, dairy, and all meat products are totally acidic when our bodies digest them. This basically means that these foods have to be banned from our diets.

Most animal foods, animal foods, and highly processed foods will have an acidic effect on the body. The best way you can help your body is to consume a diet of alkaline-forming foods.

Even if you are vegan but you only eat protein bars, you are going to wind up with an unhealthy and acidic bloodstream. An omnivore who eats many vegetables and fruits could stay alkaline and healthy.

What this is saying is our bodies have to stay in homeostasis and have a blood pH level of about 7.46 to keep our health good. This can be done by eating a diet of alkaline-producing foods that are made up of vegetables and fruits. These are also the most nutrient-dense foods, too.

There aren't any reasons to have vegan or paleo people warring about what is right and wrong with an alkaline diet.

The facts say all they need to say. You can be acidic with any diet if you eat too many acid-forming foods like sugar, animal protein, refined carbs, and fats along with too many deep-fried foods. Being an omnivore, vegetarian, or vegan is more about ethics as long as you eat foods that are alkaline.

If you would like to get and stay healthy, junk foods and animal products have to be eliminated and everything you eat has to be an alkaline food.

Chapter 8: How Toxic Foods Increase the Risk of Disease

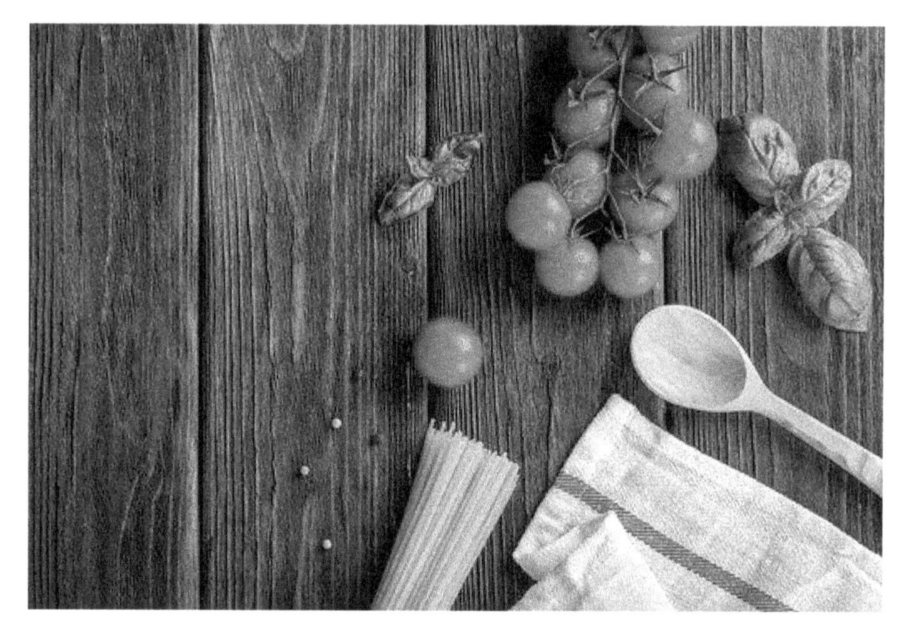

The Confusion about Acidity and Alkalinity

Some might be wondering if what we eat and drink each day can make our bodies and blood more acidic. This is extremely true. Since our bodies have a very complex nature, there is a lot more to it than just getting our bodies to an alkaline state.

Since there are parts of our bodies that have to be acidic while others, like the blood, need to be alkaline, everything we eat along with everything we drink paired with life's little stresses can all affect this outcome. Let me see if I can explain this a bit better.

Our bodies are a complex set of various systems like the lymphatic system, endocrine system, and digestive system along with the ecosystem of muscles, fluids, bones, fats, nerves, and organs.

Some of these like the stomach need to be acidic just to be able to digest foods. Our stomachs are very acidic. Our bloodstream should be a bit alkaline. Since the blood's plasma is vital to keeping the body's health systems functioning the right way, the people who favor the alkaline diet are right. We do need to consume a diet that is alkaline in order to keep our bodies healthy.

If our diets are too acidic or if we eat too many refined carbs, grains, eggs, dairy, meats, sugar, then our body's system begins breaking down and this will eventually make our blood too acidic. This is what all those experts left out when they said what we drink and eat doesn't affect our body's acidic and alkaline balance. It most certainly does. Sometimes it can cause horrible consequences.

An acidic versus alkaline body could mean the difference between sickness and health, the difference between dying early of diabetes, cancer, or heart disease or living a long and healthy life. Let's find out more about how this can happen.

Hidden Truths About the Body's pH

The alkaline and acidity levels get measured by a pH scale of 1 to 14. Our stomachs will have a pH level of one or two and this makes them very acidic. Blood, which has a pH level that is between 7.36 to 7.50 is slightly alkaline.

Our blood's pH level gets regulated by a system of buffers that work 24 / 7 to keep this narrow range of alkalinity. Because of this, most people who follow the paleo diet proclaim that you don't need to worry about anything. Just eat all the meat you want, and everything will be fine.

These paleo people tell us that our body's buffer system takes care of all this acidity. They claim that this is backed by science. If you look at your body's ecology, you will see that this idea isn't based on science. It is only a myth.

This means that the vegetarians, raw foodies, and vegans are correct. We have to eat alkaline foods to remain in optimal health. There are still most vegetarians and vegans who don't completely understand everything that is happening. Most vegetarians and vegans are too acidic and not in perfect health.

The reasons lie in the subtlety and complexity of all the organs that are involved in absorption, digestion, and elimination of all the toxins in our bodies.

Advantages

The healthiest blood pH will be in between 7.42 and 7.50. The cells can operate most efficiently at this range. Our health and life depend on our body's physiological power to keep the blood pH stable at about 7.46 through homeostasis.

This is the issue that people who deny how important alkaline foods are missing. It is the need to keep homeostasis. If your blood pH gets a bit less alkaline like below the range of 7.46 because of a breakdown in the buffer system of the body, then the body's mechanisms begin to break down, too.

How do we remain in homeostasis? We have to be sure that our body's buffering system doesn't get too overtaxed by consuming too many foods that are acidic. If the body gets too acidic, we might begin suffering from kidney stones, gall stones, osteoporosis, and other extremely undesirable health challenges.

Let's look at how fundamental pH is and how our bodies regulate the alkaline-acid balance of all its fluid every moment of every day.

Our body's pH keeps a measurement of how alkaline and acidic a liquid is. When talking about our physiology, the involved liquids are bodily fluids that can be put into two groups: the extracellular fluids like the plasma of blood and the interstitial fluids that fill the space around the tissues like the nervous system, cardiovascular system, lymphatic system, joints, etc. and the intracellular fluids that are found in our cells.

PH Scale and How to Read It

Every number on the pH scale represents a difference that is tenfold from the number above or below it. This means that a liquid that has a pH of six is ten times more acidic than something that has a pH of seven. Something that has a pH of five is one hundred times more acidic than water.

Any time we eat or drink anything, the end product of digestion and assimilation of the nutrients usually results in either an alkaline or acid-forming effect. These end products sometimes get called alkaline ash or acid ash.

Our cells also produce energy constantly. Various acids get formed and then released into the bodily fluids. These acids that are generated by our normal activities can't be avoided. If your body has to create energy in order to just survive, it produces a constant acid supply.

There are two things that can disrupt our body's pH: the acids we generate by doing regular metabolic activities and the alkaline or acid-forming effects of liquids and foods.

Plus, stress could affect the acid levels in the body because we normally don't digest food properly if we are on the go constantly and are stressed. Fortunately, our bodies have three mechanisms to help prevent these things from shifting our blood's pH out of the optimal range.

Body's Buffer

Our bodies do have a buffer system of carbonic acids, a phosphate buffer system, and a protein buffer system. Plus, we buffer ourselves when we exhale carbon dioxide and by getting rid of hydrogen through the kidneys.

It is because of these facts that experts say that certain foods can't have any negative effects on our health by affecting the acidity alkaline balance. Their main argument is our body's buffering system can take care of anything that we decide to eat.

This is so false that it isn't even funny. When you eat junk food that contains too many refined carbs, sugars, and animal fats, the buffering system gets overloaded and can't protect the blood from getting too acidic. This means our bodies can't maintain homeostasis. This is when we begin getting sick.

If our bodies are constantly exposed to huge quantities of liquids and foods that form acids, your body will call on its calcium phosphate reserves to give your phosphate buffer system everything it needs to neutralize the acids in your diet. With time, this might lead to weaknesses in your teeth and bones.

Consuming a diet of acid-forming foods could increase the risk of developing kidney stones. One other common effect of a diet rich in acidic foods along with stress is acid-reflux. It is in your best interest not to overtax your body's buffering system by consuming foods that produce alkaline.

Impacts of Foods on Urine and Blood pH

Nourishments desert an acid or alkaline debris. Acid debris contains phosphate and sulfur. Chemical waste contains calcium, magnesium, and potassium.

Specific nutritional categories are viewed as acidic, nonpartisan, or alkaline.

Acidic: Meats, fish, dairy, eggs, grains, and liquor.

Neutral: Fats, starches, and sugars.

Alkaline: Fruits, vegetables, nuts, and vegetables.

Urine pH

Nourishments you eat change the pH of your pee. If you have a green smoothie for breakfast, your pee, in a couple of hours, will be more alkaline than if you had bacon and eggs. For somebody on an alkaline diet, pee pH can be effectively checked and may even give moment delight. Sadly, pee pH is neither a decent pointer of the general pH of the body, nor is it a suitable marker of public health.

Blood pH

The nourishments you eat don't change your blood pH. At the point when you eat something with acid debris like protein, the acids created are immediately killed by bicarbonate particles in the blood. This response produces carbon dioxide, which is breathed out through the lungs, and salts, which are discharged by the kidneys in your pee. During the procedure of discharge, the kidneys produce new bicarbonate particles, which are come back to the blood to supplant the bicarbonate that was at first used to kill the acid. This makes a reasonable cycle wherein the body can keep up the pH of the blood inside a tight range.

In this way, as long as your kidneys are working typically, your blood pH won't be impacted by the nourishments you eat, regardless of whether they are acidic or alkaline. The case that eating alkaline nourishments will make your body or blood pH progressively alkaline isn't valid.

Acidic Diet and Cancer

The individuals who advocate an alkaline diet guarantee that it can fix cancer since cancer can just develop in an acidic domain. By eating an alkaline diet, cancer cells can't develop; however, bite the dust. This speculation is exceptionally defective. Cancer is flawlessly equipped for developing in an alkaline situation. Cancer develops in healthy body tissue, which has a somewhat alkaline pH of 7.4. Numerous analyses have affirmed this by effectively developing cancer cells in an alkaline domain.

Be that as it may, cancer cells do become quicker with acidity. When a tumor begins to create, it makes its very own acidic condition by separating glucose and decreasing flow. Along these lines, it isn't the acidic condition that causes cancer, yet cancer that causes the acidic disease. Significantly all the more fascinating is a recent report by the National Cancer Institute, which utilizes nutrient C (ascorbic acid) to treat cancer. They found that by directing pharmacologic portions intravenously, ascorbic acid effectively murdered cancer cells without hurting healthy cells. This is another case of cancer cells being powerless against acidity, instead of alkalinity.

To put it plainly, there is no logical connection between eating an acidic diet and cancer. Cancer cells can develop in both acidic and alkaline conditions.

Acidic Diet and Osteoporosis

Osteoporosis is a progressive bone disease described by a decline in bone mineral substance, prompting brought down the bone thickness and quality and greater danger of a messed-up bone. Advocates of the alkaline diet accept that to keep up a steady blood pH, the body takes alkaline minerals like calcium from the unresolved issues the acids from acidic food. As examined over, this is in no way, shape, or form genuine. The kidneys and the respiratory framework are answerable for managing blood pH, not the bones.

Numerous examinations have indicated that expanding creature protein admission is sure for bone digestion as it builds calcium maintenance and actuates IGF-1 (insulin-like development factor-1) that animates bone recovery. In this manner, the speculation that an acidic diet causes bone loss isn't upheld by science.

Acidic Diet and Muscle Wasting

Backers of the alkaline diet accept that to dispense with overabundance acid brought about by acidic food, the kidneys will take amino acids (building squares of protein) from muscle tissues, prompting muscle loss. The proposed system is like the one causing osteoporosis. As examined, blood pH is controlled by the kidneys and the lungs, not the muscles. Thus, acidic nourishments like meats, dairy, and eggs don't cause muscle loss. Indeed, they are complete dietary proteins that will bolster muscle fix and help anticipate muscle squandering.

What Did Our Ancestors Eat?

Various investigations have inspected whether our pre-farming predecessors ate net acidic or net alkaline diets. Interestingly, they found that a portion of the tracker gatherers ate net acid-framing foods, while the other half ate profit alkaline-shaping diets. Acid-framing meals were progressively regular as individuals moved further north of the equator. The less approachable the earth, the more creature proteins they ate. In progressively tropical conditions where foods grown from the ground were plenteous, their diet turned out to be increasingly alkaline.

The facts confirm that numerous individuals who have changed to an alkaline diet see massive health enhancements. In any case, do remember that different reasons might be grinding away:

Most of us don't eat enough vegetables and natural products. As indicated by the Center for Disease and Prevention, just 9% of Americans eat enough vegetables and 13% enough natural products. If you change to an alkaline diet, you are consequently eating more vegetables and organic products. They are wealthy in phytochemicals, cancer prevention agents, and fiber, which are essential to excellent health. At the point when you eat more vegetables and natural products, you are presumably eating less handled nourishments as well.

Eating less dairy and eggs will profit the individuals who are lactose-bigoted or have a nourishment affectability to eggs, which is relatively healthy among the all-inclusive community.

Eating fewer grains will profit the individuals who are gluten-delicate or have broken gut or an immune system disease.

Alkaline Water

One final point worth referencing is that numerous individuals accept that drinking alkaline water (pH of 9.5 versus pure water's pH of 7.0.) is healthier dependent on comparable thinking as the alkaline diet. At any rate, it isn't valid. Water that is too alkaline can be contrary to your health and lead to wholesome disequilibrium.

On the off chance that you drink alkaline water regularly, it will kill your stomach acid and raise the alkalinity of your stomach. After some time, it will impede your capacity to process nourishment and assimilate supplements and minerals. With less acidity in the stomach, it will likewise open the entryway for microscopic organisms and parasites to get into your small digestive system. Most importantly, alkaline water isn't a response to excellent health. Try not to be tricked by showcasing contrivances. Instead, put resources into a decent water filtration framework for your home. Clean, separated water is as yet the best water for your body.

At the point when you decide to eat an alkaline diet, you are eating nourishments that are fundamentally the same as what man was intended to eat. If you take a gander at what our progenitors ate, you will discover a diet wealthy in new natural products, vegetables, vegetables, nuts, and fish. Shockingly, man's diet today is much of the time loaded with nourishments that are high in unhealthy fats, salt, cholesterol, and acidifying food sources.

How Our Diet Changed

Albeit a few people believe that man's diet changed as of late, the move from or to an excellent extent alkaline diet to an acid diet started a considerable number of years back. Our unique diet comprised of scavenged natural products, nuts, and vegetables; alongside whatever meat could be gotten. When man began to develop his very own nourishment, things began to change. Grains turned into a well-known diet decision, particularly after the advancement of stone instruments. When creatures were trained, there were dairy items added to the diet, alongside an extra measure of meat. Salt started to be included, alongside sugar. The final product was a diet that was still a lot healthier than what numerous individuals eat today. However, the move from alkaline to acid had started.

Late Dietary Changes

It's a well-known fact that our advanced diet comprises of numerous nourishments which are not healthy for us. An excessive amount of shoddy nourishment and "inexpensive food" has diminished the nature of our menu. Heftiness has become the standard and alongside it a higher rate of diseases, for example, diabetes, coronary disease, and cancer. On the off chance that you need to improve your health and lessen the danger of numerous diseases, an alkaline diet can help recover your body to nuts and bolts.

At the point when nourishments are eaten and processed, they produce either an acidifying or alkalizing impact inside the body. A few people get confounded because the real pH of the nourishment itself doesn't have anything to do with the effects of the food once it is processed. At the point when progressively alkaline nourishments are devoured, the body can turn out to be marginally alkaline rather than acid. Preferably, the blood pH level ought to be somewhere in the range of 7.35 and 7.45. Nourishments, for example, organic citrus products, soy items, homemade leafy foods, wild rice, almonds, and regular sugars, for instance, Stevia are generally significant alkaline nourishment decisions.

There are numerous advantages to moving your eating designs from acid to alkaline. At the point when the body is kept somewhat alkaline, it is less helpless to disease. It's simpler to shed pounds or keep up a healthy weight level on an alkaline diet. A great many people experience an expansion in their energy level, just as a decreasing of uneasiness and fractiousness once they start eating increasingly caustic nourishments. Mucous creation is diminished, and the nasal clog is decreased, making it simpler to breathe. Hypersensitivities are much of the time mitigated because of an alkaline diet. The body is additionally less helpless to diseases, for example, cancer and diabetes. A great many people find that they simply feel good, with an expanded feeling of health and prosperity, when they endeavor to hold fast to an alkaline diet.

Picking Alkaline Diets Is the Only Way to Live a Healthy Lifestyle

The low carbohydrate and high protein diets doing the rounds nowadays are a solicitation to poor health. All competitors realize that if a fit body is to be kept up, one should avoid such diets. In addition to the fact that they result in extreme weariness are where weight the executives are concerned. Picking alkaline foods is the best way to carry on with a healthy life just as shed those additional pounds.

Alkaline diets expect one to pursue a way of direct life inverse of the high protein low carb diets. The high protein diets leave the individual tailing it exhausted and tired. It is for the individuals who have a dormant existence and need to shed some weight. In any case, the weight that is lost returns on when one stops the diet. With alkaline foods, this isn't the situation. The menus can be joined into one's lifestyle, and within days the outcomes start to show. They expect one to eat around 80 % alkalizing nourishments to keep up the alkaline ph. of the body to 7.4. High protein diets will, in general, make the ph. of the body acidic instead of its standard alkaline tilt at the point when the body ph. becomes acidic. It pulls in all sicknesses and exhausts one of energy — an acidic ph.

Additionally, brings about quick degeneration of the human body cells. That prompts an abbreviated life. One should avoid these accident diets and take a gander at accomplishing health and energy by following alkaline foods.

Alkaline diets lead to body ph. It is keeping up its chemical nature. The different body capacities are completed quickly, and the insusceptible arrangement of the body remains solid. Under these conditions, one feels enthusiastic rather than feeling exhausted. Additionally, the weight shed like this stays off, and in particular, the body doesn't fall debilitated. As such, they help repulse diseases instead of high protein diets, which appear to pull in them. These plans are likewise generally excellent for those experiencing interminable diseases like joint pain, cancer, headaches, sinusitis, and osteoporosis. Following such a system while taking prescription helps fend these diseases off from the root.

Alkaline diets generally comprise of foods grown from the ground. One should attempt to expend green vegetables and sweet natural products with the goal that they make up around 70 to 80 percent of their all-out nourishment admission. Lemons and melons ought to likewise be eaten. Almonds, nectar, and olive oil are additionally high on the rundown of nourishments to be expended for following alkaline diets. Meats and fats ought to stay away from. All nourishments that are acidifying like espresso, liquor, pork, and even certain vegetables like cooked spinach ought not to shape over 20% of one's diet. Alkaline water is additionally an unquestionable requirement for everybody needing to improve their diet. At any rate, 6 to 8 glasses of alkaline water can do wonders for your body purifying. Prepared nourishment is all acidic and high on weight picking up substances, thus ought to be kept away from. Drinks like soft drinks are profoundly acidic and ought not to be expended by any stretch of the imagination. It takes 32 glasses of water to adjust one glass of pop. Alkaline diets are for everybody. Every last one of us should quit manhandling our bodies and take a gander at a healthy and long life by making alkaline diets a piece of our way of life.

The Benefits of Dr. Sebi's Medicine

He created this diet for anybody who wants to prevent or cure any disease naturally. It can also improve your overall health without using chemical medications.

Dr. Sebi's theory is that all diseases are caused because of too much mucus building up in a specific area of the body. When you have too much mucus in your lungs, you get pneumonia. If you have too much mucus in your pancreas, it causes diabetes.

He believes that any disease won't be able to exist in an environment that is alkaline but can happen if your body is too acidic.

If you can follow this diet very strictly while using his supplements, you will be able to restore your body to a healthy alkaline state while detoxifying your body.

Many people claim that his diet improved their health by using his compounds and the herbal approach to heal the body worked better than any medical approach ever did. You can find many of his thoughts about herbal therapy and nutritional compounds on YouTube that help promote and teach healthy living long after his death.

His diet does offer many health benefits. The main one is it can promote weight loss because it restricts processed foods and you will be eating more plant-based, unprocessed meals. This diet is full of whole fruits and vegetables that are full of plant compounds, minerals, vitamins, and fiber.

Diets that are rich in fruits and vegetables are associated with oxidative stress and reduced inflammation along with protecting you against most diseases.

Meatless diets have been linked to lower risks of heart disease and obesity. It also encourages foods that are high in fiber and low in calories. Regularly consuming fruits and vegetables can help protect your body against diseases and reduce inflammation.

If you can switch from your normal diet that is full of fast foods, saturated fats, refined sugars, and grains to Dr. Sebi's diet could actually help you lose some weight. Increasing your intake of whole grains, vegetables, and fruits while getting rid of pork and beef can decrease your risk of elevated cholesterol, high blood pressure, Type 2 diabetes, heart disease, and cancer. Most people eat way too much sodium and this diet can drastically lower this amount. This, in turn, can help you lower your blood pressure, and this reduces your risk of heart disease and stroke.

In one study people who ate seven servings of fruits and vegetables each day had between a 25 and 31 percent lower chances of heart disease and cancer.

Most Americans don't eat enough produce. During 2017 it was reported that between 9.3 and 12.2 percent met all their recommended daily intake of fruits and vegetables.

Dr. Sebi's diet encourages eating healthy fats like plant oils, seeds, and nuts along with whole grain that is rich in fiber. These foods have a lower risk of developing heart disease.

Any diet that limits processed foods can help you have a better quality of diet.

Food is Powerful

After seeing all the food documentaries and getting all the GMO warnings and all the chicken farms and slaughterhouses being exposed, we are faced with one question: "Could the decline of our health and rise of diseases finally convince urban and poor communities to turn to a plant-based diet?"

Poor people suffer from one major health crisis: a horrible diet.

It is devastating when families have to bury family members especially when they are always the life of the party at reunions. These people love eating comfort foods like mac and cheese, collard greens, barbecue ribs, and fried chicken. Everybody loves eating comfort foods. It's a way to enjoy ourselves. We've watched family members die from heart disease, strokes, diabetes, and cancer. We eat the foods that our elders pass down to us. Some family members suffer from hypertension while others have to have dialysis weekly because they are suffering from kidney failure. These people die at young ages and leave behind children and grieving spouses. It is these moments that help you realize that some "traditions" have to be done away with.

Maybe it is time for you to do some research on alkaline and plant-based diets.

There have been many people who have actually healed themselves by following Dr. Sebi's diet while others have reversed some serious medical conditions. After doing your research, you might realize that there has been a lot of misleading information and confusion within the food industry. Pigs, cows, and chickens are being tortured, tampered with, and then tossed on our plates. We eat these animals and we are digesting all their agony and angst. If some of our late relatives had this information, they could have made different choices and lived a long life.

Many people have written cookbooks about the alkaline diet and they have healed themselves by changing the way they eat. Some thought they had been living a healthy lifestyle but were diagnosed with diseases, nonetheless.

Upon doing more research, they realized that food plays a larger role in our lives other than just keeping us from being hungry. Then they dug deeper and realized that the food industry has been lying to us for years about how our foods are packaged.

The more they researched, they figured out the meat market is a huge money-making industry and fills our heads with a lot of propaganda. Our bodies are electric, and they need food just like a car needs a battery. It needs things that will spark energy into it.

When we eat dead animals that don't have any living cells, what will it do to our bodies? NOTHING. It just makes our bodies fight to get rid of it since it doesn't do anything. Putting this in our bodies just makes them have to work harder to get fuel.

After doing more research about Dr. Sebi, they realized that his regimen could actually help. They didn't just write a cookbook about his diet, they actually did a 30-day regimen and within one week, their problems began to go away.

One particular author was diagnosed with carpal tunnel and after following Dr. Sebi's diet for one week, her carpal tunnel was better because her body had gotten rid of its excess mucus.

Their largest challenge was finding the right food in supermarkets. Finding the vegetables, plants, and grains that weren't hybrid can be difficult. Then they had to figure out how to create recipes that were cost-effective and simple. There are many people who don't eat many fruits and vegetables because they are expensive. Junk food, meats, processed foods are cheaper and more readily available.

Deciding to create a cookbook with simple easy recipes that can make people feel full plus was easy on the wallet wasn't a hard decision to make. Most people don't even think about questioning the food industry about how their food is created or where the food comes from.

Social media makes it possible to call out these industries on their lies and propaganda. We don't have to continue thinking we have to drink milk in order to have strong bones because you can get that through plant-based foods. People are beginning to question all this misinformation we have been bombarded with for years. They no longer have to believe all the lies the dairy and meat companies have fed us for years.

The reasons why urban communities have a hard time learning how to eat healthier:

Tradition

These traditions have been fed to us since our birth. Our society promotes junk food daily and it is going to take strong people to break this tradition of the culture and society they are in.

Addiction and habit

Habits are extremely hard to break. Most of the foods we eat that are processed are full of chemicals that make us dependent on them. It isn't any different than asking a smoker to put down their cigarettes.

Not Enough Information

When the meat and dairy industries have a lot of control over our governments, they won't be any concern or information for the people. Money is worth more than the truth. Most of the brown communities suffer from diseases such as obesity, high blood pressure, heart disease, diabetes, and asthma. All of these diseases can be totally reversed and healed by picking foods that are healthier like fresh vegetables and fruits, drinking water, meditating, and exercising.

Chapter 9: Supplements to Take Daily

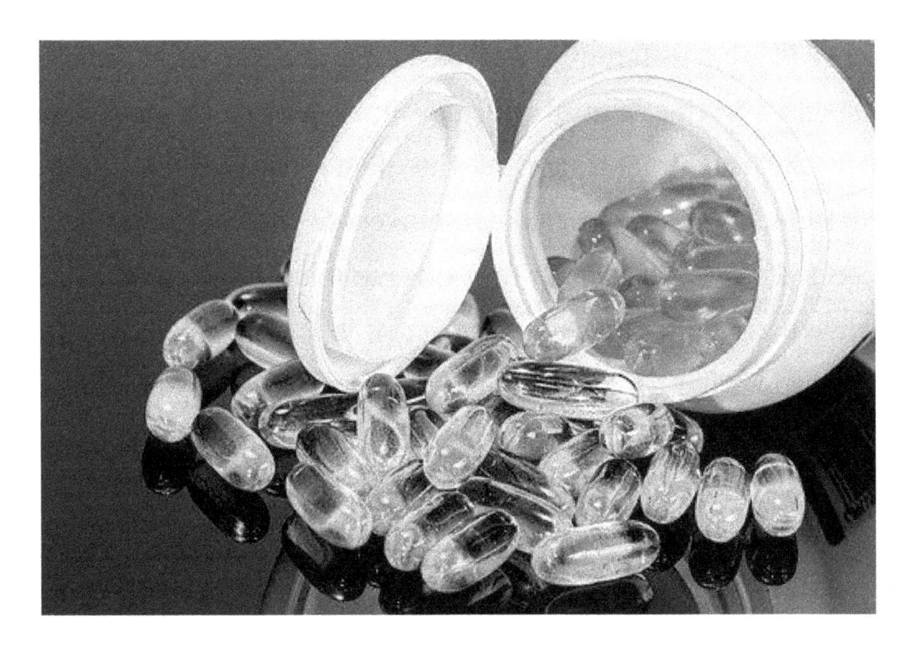

Along with the restrictive diet, you have to buy Dr. Sebi's original blend of supplements for effective disease curing therapy and weight loss. You can buy the supplements from Dr. Sebi's food cell website. Although the curing properties of these compounds were debunked a long time ago, the compounds' effectiveness in weight loss has still not been proven. There is no scientific study that has given definitive evidence that these chemicals/products do what they claim. Regardless, many of Dr. Sebi's clients and followers still believe that they are very beneficial and are irreplaceable.

What are the Supplements Made Of?

They are made by all organic and natural ingredients and blended with the knowledge of Dr. Sebi. They mostly contain seaweed and different types of herbs and algae. It mostly dispenses in the form of capsules and needs to be consumed daily by the practitioner of the diet. Some of Dr. Sebi's mixtures or products can contain exotic flowers and other pieces of plants. They can be a diverse mixture or consist of a single ingredient entirely. However, it is important to say that when you order a set of the products, many bottles are labeled that they contain some undisclosed ingredient not mentioned previously. This can be a serious hazard if you find yourself allergic to different substances or get sensitive reactions easily.

Are Supplements Enough?

The diet has no nutritional or individual nutrient-based guidance. It doesn't tell us how to maintain normal levels of all the basic nutrients, which include proteins, fats, and other components of a balanced diet. One of the major concerns in any plant-based diet is malnutrition development from protein deficiency. Unlike vegetarian or vegan dieting, this diet restricts not only the meat of any animal-source but also some seeds, nuts, grains, and soy products. These ingredients are plant-based alternative foods to replenish protein supply. To get good amounts of protein and also other components this diet limits, you need to opt for protein supplements or any other kind of supplements that you may think is needed other than the ones provided by Dr. Sebi's food cell.

Are They Worth the Expense?

Some products available in Dr. Sebi's food cell are too expensive for it to be a part of an everyday regiment for most people. Getting a bottle of their products can cost up to $30 per bottle, and it is instructed that you have to take a pill each day. There have been no proven studies showing that the products even work, and on top of that, they sell the products with strict rules and great fare. Buying vegetables and whole foods are already very pricey as it is in this day and age for it to be capped by more expenses. For an effective weight loss routine, you don't need these pills to help you reach your weight loss goals. The diet itself is low enough in calories that you will see weight loss regardless.

Must-Have Dr. Sebi Products

To help you out, we are going to look at the five Dr. Sebi products that you must start with. After you have become more used to Dr. Sebi's diet and products, you can start to increase the number of supplements you take or change them to something that supports your body the best.

Viento

Viento is a powerful product that helps to improve the entire body, which includes cleansing the lymphatic system, central nervous system, respiratory system, kidneys, and brain. The key ingredient of viento is the chaparral, which is a powerful antioxidant, but that's not the only this it contains.

Sapo is often used to help anorexia, worms, inflammation, swelling, indigestion, and liver disorders. It is also sometimes used as a uterine tonic.

Hombre Grande is often used to help with dyspepsia, anorexia, nematode infestation, pediculosis, and antonic dyspepsia with loss of appetite.

Contribo has been used to treat oxytocic, diaphoretic, stimulant, sterility, menstrual irregularities, snake bites, and leprosy. It also acts as an immune enhancer. It can also stimulate the action of the white blood cells.

Chaparral has been used to help itching, tetanus, piles, chest complaints, kidney disorders, indigestion, delayed menses, healing wounds, lumbago, skin disorders, arthritis, rheumatism, and sexually transmitted diseases.

Valraiana is often used to treat seizures, convulsions, tension headaches, multiple sclerosis, and works as a calmative, antispasmodic, and stimulating tonic and nervine.

Irish sea moss is often used to nourish the body due to its high mineral content. It can also help with bladder and kidney irritation, stomach ulcers, gastritis, lung problems, irritating coughs, digestive issues, and anti-viral.

Bromide Plus Capsules or Powder

You can take bromide plus as a pill or use the powder to make a tea. The powder is more commonly used because it can be mixed into shakes as well as made into a tea. The ingredients help to nourish the thyroid gland and bones. It helps the digestive system as a whole and also helps the respiratory and pulmonary systems.

The Irish sea moss contained in the bromide plus powder is a great source of minerals. It has historically been used to treat dry coughs, pulmonary tuberculosis, inflammation of the bladder and kidneys, bronchitis, and respiratory disorders. It can be helpful for people who suffer from wasting health conditions and need to gain weight. It also helps if you have an inflammation of the alimentary canal, and also protects the gastrointestinal system.

Bladderwrack is a seaweed that is full of micronutrients, mainly copper, zinc, silicon, sulphur, manganese, sodium, and iodine. It helps the endocrine gland and stimulates the circulation in the lymphatic system. It helps with hypothyroidism and helps aid in weight loss. It is also a mild diuretic.

Bio Ferro Tonic

This tonic is great for increasing your energy levels without feeling over-stimulated or hyperactive. It is meant to help improve every bodily system because if its iron content.

The yellow dock root is high in iron and is recommended for people who have chronic skin diseases or blood disorders. We have to have iron in order for our bodies to function properly. Every single cell in our body contains iron.

Burdock root is great for cleansing the body. It is very helpful for the kidneys because it contains tannins that can help with arthritis, ulcers, gout, kidney damage, and upset stomach. In China, they use it to help sterility, and in India, it is used for cancer.

Elderberry is great for the immune system and helps prevent the common cold. It also encourages toxins to be eliminated. It is also an anti-inflammatory and can help to lower your cholesterol levels. This berry can also help to keep candida under control.

Cocolmeca is a favorite for men because it works a lot like Viagra. It comes from the rainforests of Belize where they would boil it and give it to the men. It has a lot of benefits for women as well, such as increased vitality.

Sarsparilla has been historically used to treat leprosy, gonorrhea, and syphilis. It is also great for overall wellness and works as an anti-inflammatory. It is especially helpful for the cells in the liver.

Lymphalin

Lymphalin works to remove all of the calcification in the body. It is a mineral gold, which is important for the body and helps the body to break up calcification.

Hydrangea, or hortensia, in the supplement helps with cystitis, phosphaturia, stony deposits, calcium oxalate deposits, mucus irritation of the bladder, and chronic gleet. It can also relieve backaches that are caused by kidney problems, as well as rheumatism, arteriosclerosis, and arthritis.

Cascar sagrada, or pushiana, is great for relieving bad breath, healing cirrhosis, assisting in liver function, relieving congestion in the gall and liver duct, and habitual constipation.

Red clover helps people who have wasting diseases, such as rickets, as well as whooping cough, and spasmodic affections.

Palo mulato is often used as an antiseptic diuretic. It can also help with urinary tract infections, sunburns, sunstroke, skin sores, rashes, measles, insect bites, flu, fevers, blood cleansing, colds, nephritis, diarrhea, and calculus.

Chelation 2

Chelation 2 is meant to help detoxify the mucus membranes throughout the body. It helps to remove mucus, acids, and toxins while also providing the body with mineral nourishment that it needs during the cleansing process. It will also help to increase your daily bowel movement.

Cascara sagrada has a very long history of use in the Native American culture where it has been used as an herbal laxative and to support digestive health. It is full of phytochemicals that work as stimulant laxatives. It is a tonic for the digestive system. It causes a cascade of things to happen within the body to get it ready for the digestive process. It is also an anti-microbial and anti-parasitic.

Prodigiosa is a flowering plant that has long been used to help lower high blood sugar levels for type 2 diabetics, motivate the digestion of fats in the gallbladder, and it helps to improve digestion. In some people, it can also help or prevent cataracts.

Pao Pereira is a native tree to South America. It has historically been used as a sexual stimulant, and used to treat cancer, liver pain, fever, constipation, digestive disorders, and malaria.

Rhubarb is a root vegetable that is high in magnesium, dietary fiber, manganese, potassium, calcium, vitamin K, and vitamin C. It can help to lower cholesterol levels and is a great source of antioxidants.

Chapter 10: Dr. Sebi Approved Recipes

Breakfast

Quinoa Porridge

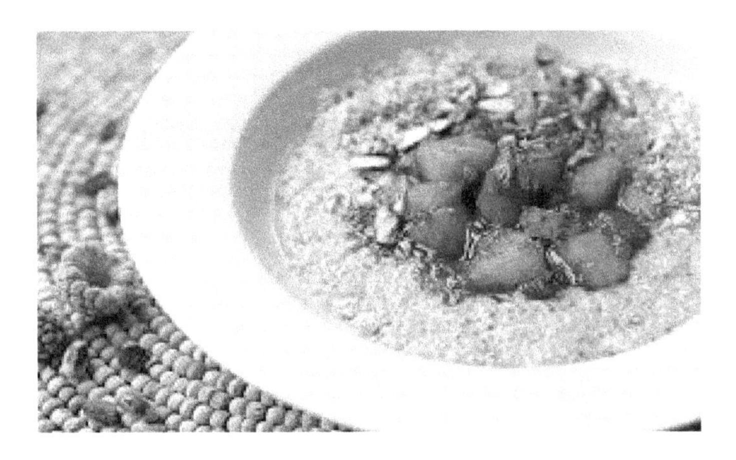

Preparation Time: 5 minutes

Cooking Time: 25 minutes

Servings: 2

Ingredients:

2 cups coconut milk

1 cup rinsed quinoa

1/8 tsp. ground cinnamon

1 cup fresh blueberries

Directions:

In a saucepan, boil the coconut milk over high heat.

Add the quinoa to the milk then bring the mixture to a boil.

You then let it simmer for 15 minutes on medium heat until the milk is reduced.

Add the cinnamon then mix it properly in the saucepan.

Cover the saucepan and cook for at least 8 minutes until the milk is completely absorbed.

Add in the blueberries then cook for 30 more seconds.

Serve.

Zucchini Bread Pancakes

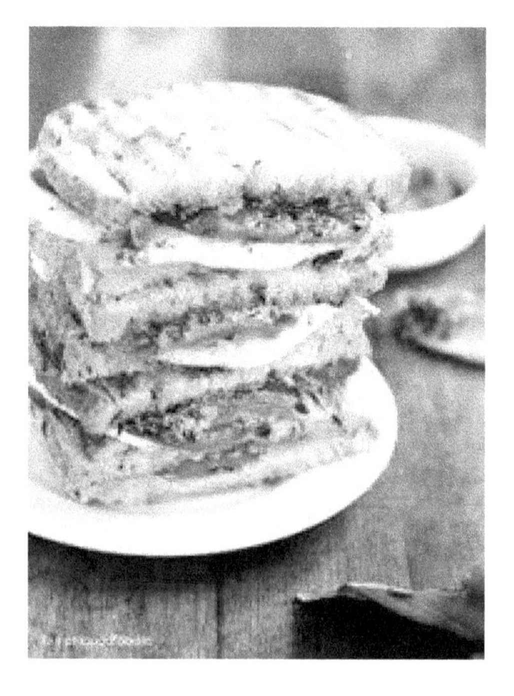

Preparation Time: 5 minutes

Cooking Time: 20 minutes

Servings: 2

Ingredients:

2 cups spelt or kamut flour

2 tbsp date sugar

1/4 cup mashed burro banana

1 cup finely shredded zucchini

2 cups homemade walnut milk

1/2 cup chopped walnuts

1 tbsp grapeseed oil

Directions:

In a large bowl, whisk flour and date sugar.

Pour in walnut milk and mashed burro banana. Stir until just combined, making sure to scrape the bottom of the bowl so there are no pockets of dry mix. Stir in shredded zucchini and walnuts.

Heat grapeseed oil in a griddle or skillet over medium high heat.

Pour batter onto the griddle to make your pancakes. Cook 4 – 5 minutes on each side.

Serve with agave syrup and enjoy!

Basil Avocado Pasta Salad

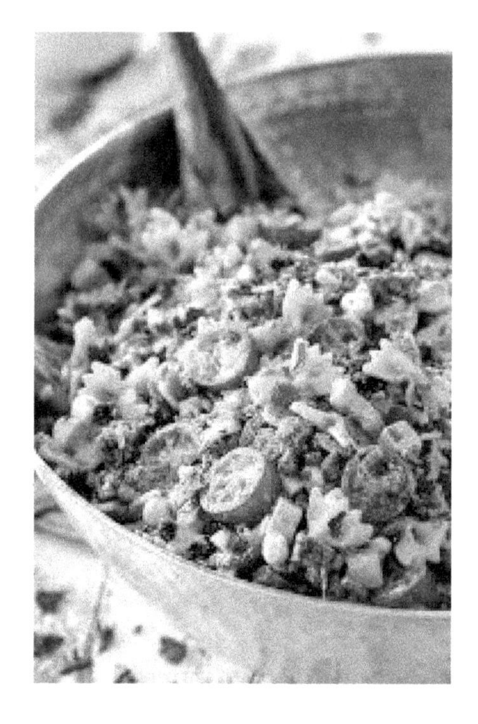

Preparation Time: 5 minutes

Cooking Time: 30 minutes

Servings: 2

Ingredients:

1 avocado, chopped

1 cup fresh basil, chopped

1-pint cherry tomatoes halved

1 tbsp key lime juice

1 tsp agave syrup

1/4 cup olive oil

4 cups cooked spelt pasta

Directions:

Place cooked pasta in a large bowl.

Add avocado, basil and tomatoes and stir until ingredients are thoroughly mixed.

In a small mixing bowl, whisk together oil, lime juice, agave syrup, and sea salt. Pour over pasta and stir to combine.

Wakame Salad

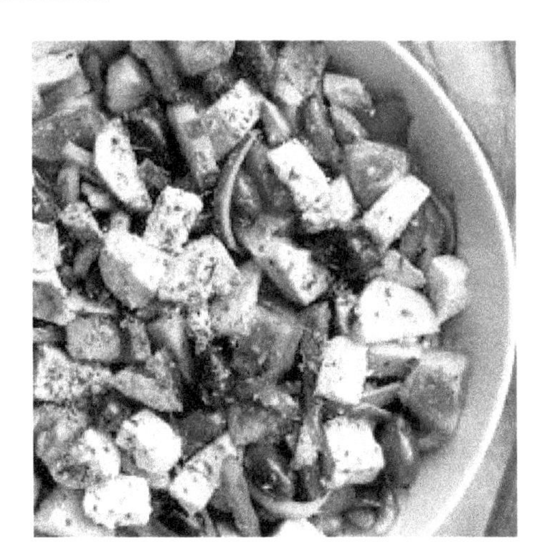

Preparation Time: 5 minutes

Cooking Time: 40 minutes

Servings: 2

Ingredients:

2 cups wakame stems

1 tsp onion powder

1 tsp ginger

1 tbsp red bell pepper

1 tbsp sesame seeds

1 tbsp key lime juice

1 tbsp agave syrup

1 tbsp sesame oil

Directions:

Soak wakame stems for 5-10 minutes and drain.

In a mixing bowl, combine sesame oil, agave syrup, key lime juice, onion powder, and ginger. Whisk thoroughly.

Place wakame and bell pepper in a serving dish. Pour dressing on top.

Sprinkle with sesame seeds and enjoy!

Grilled Romaine Lettuce Salad

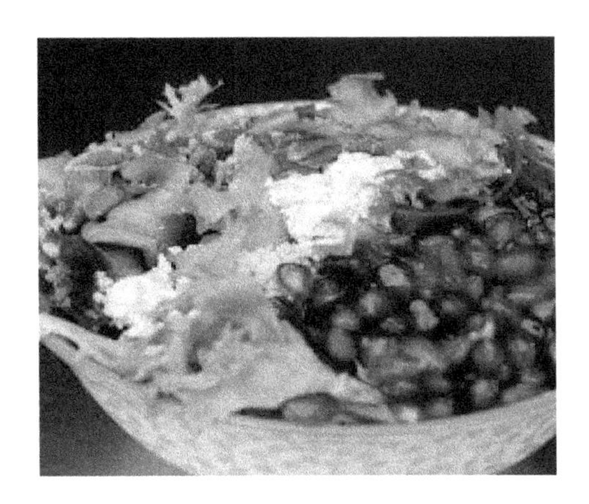

Preparation Time: 5 minutes

Cooking Time: 30 minutes

Servings: 2

Ingredients:

4 small heads romaine lettuce, rinsed

1 tbsp red onion, chopped finely

1 tbsp key lime juice

Onion powder, to taste

1 tbsp fresh basil, chopped

Sea salt and cayenne pepper, to taste

4 tbsp olive oil

1 tbsp agave syrup

Directions:

Place lettuce halves cut side down in a large nonstick pan. Don't add any oil. Check the color of the lettuce by turning them. Make sure the lettuce is browned on both sides.

Take the pan off the heat and allow lettuce to cool on a large platter.

For dressing, combine red onion with olive oil, agave syrup, key lime juice and fresh basil in a small mixing bowl. Add salt and cayenne pepper to taste. Whisk well to combine.

Transfer grilled lettuce onto a serving dish and drizzle with the dressing. Enjoy!

Dandelion Strawberry Salad

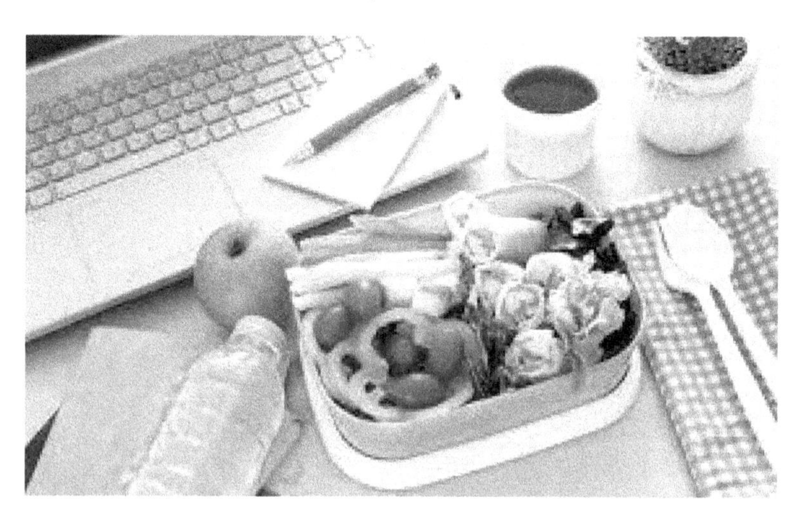

Preparation Time: 5 minutes

Cooking Time: 30 minutes

Servings: 2

Ingredients:

2 tbsp grapeseed oil

1 medium red onion, sliced

10 ripe strawberries, sliced

2 tbsp key lime juice

4 cups dandelion greens

Sea salt to taste

Directions:

Warm grapeseed oil over medium heat in a 12-inch nonstick frying pan. Add sliced onions along with a good pinch of sea salt. Cook, stirring often, until onions are soft, lightly brown, and reduced to about 1/3 of raw volume.

In a small bowl, toss strawberry slices with 1 tsp of key lime juice. Wash dandelion greens and cut into bite-sized pieces if you like.

When the onions are nearly done, add the remaining key lime juice to the pan and continue cooking until it has thickened to coat the onions, a minute or two. Remove onions from heat.

In a salad bowl, combine the greens, onions and strawberries with all their juices. Sprinkle with sea salt.

Hydrating Smoothie

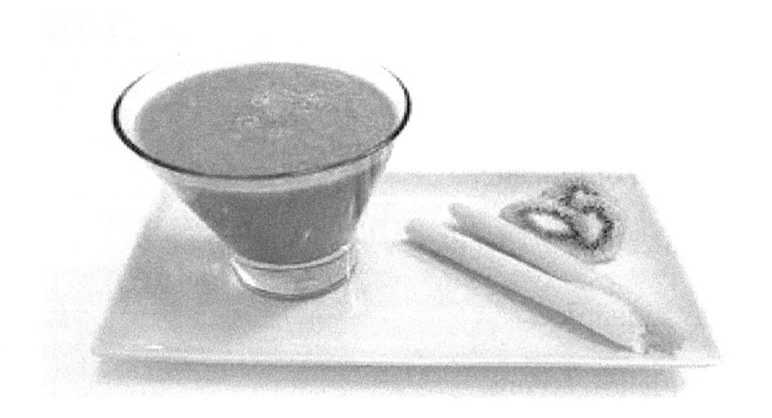

Preparation Time: 5 minutes

Cooking Time: 0 minutes

Servings: 2

Ingredients:

1 cup strawberries

1 cup watermelon chunks

1 cup soft jelly coconut water

1 tbsp date sugar

Directions:

Blend all ingredients together and enjoy!

Juicy Portobello Burgers

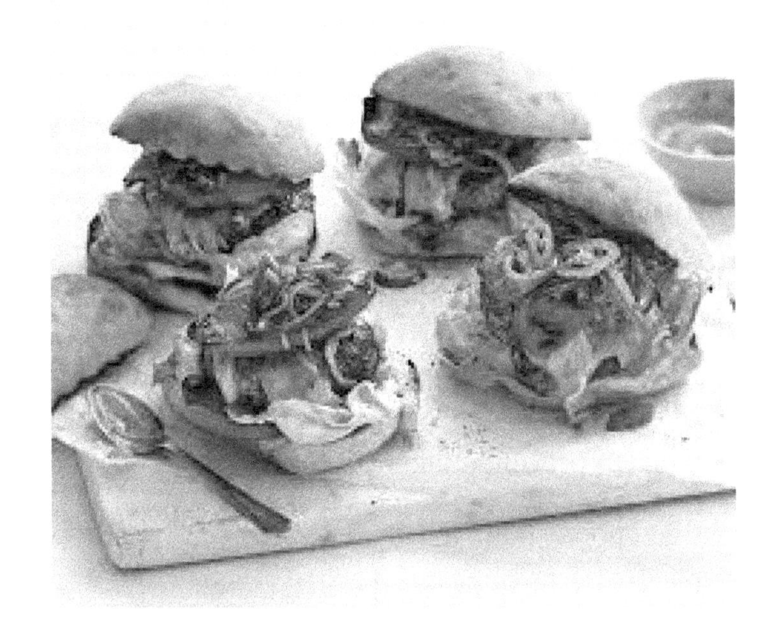

Preparation Time: 5 minutes

Cooking Time: 20 minutes

Servings: 2

Ingredients:

2 large portobello mushroom caps

3 tbsp olive oil

2 tsp dried basil

1 tsp dried oregano

1/2 tsp Cayenne pepper

1 tomato sliced

1 avocado sliced

1 cup purslane

Directions:

Slice the mushroom stems off and slice off about 1/2" of the mushroom top (as if slicing a bun).

Combine olive oil, onion powder, basil, oregano, and Cayenne pepper in a small bowl and mix well.

Place mushroom caps on a cookie sheet with foil and a little grapeseed oil (to prevent sticking).

With a large spoon, pour marinade over each mushroom cap and allow to sit about 10 mins.

Preheat oven to 425°F and bake mushrooms for about 10 mins, check the level of preparedness before flipping them to bake another 10 mins.

Place the bottom of the mushroom cap on a plate – add your choice of toppings – and top with the top portion of the baked mushroom cap.

Classic Homemade Hummus

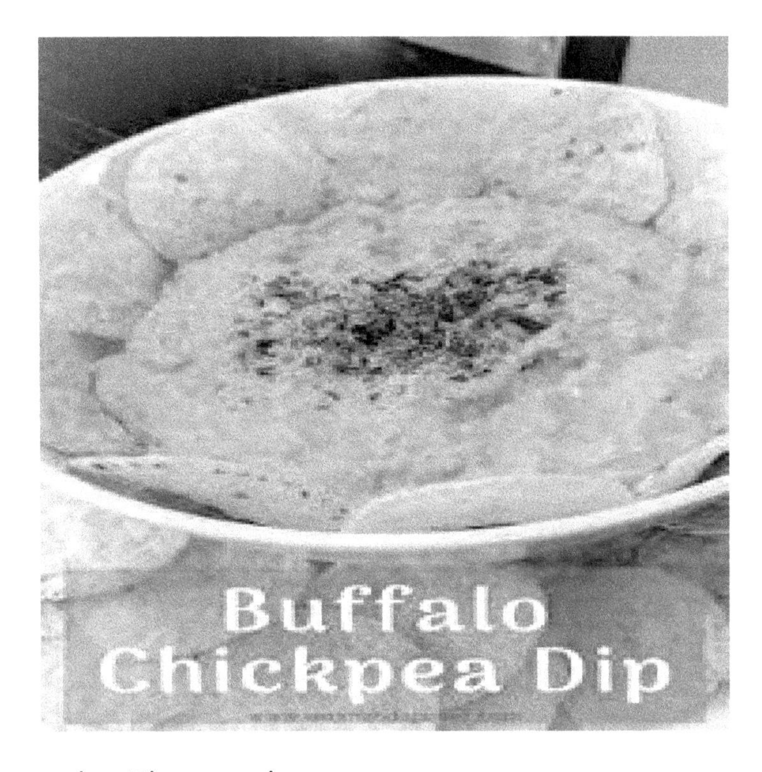

Preparation Time: 5 minutes

Cooking Time: 30 minutes

Servings: 2

Ingredients:

1 cup cooked chickpeas

1/3 cup homemade tahini butter

2 tbsp olive oil

2 tbsp key lime juice

A dash of onion powder

Sea salt, to taste

Directions:

Blend all the ingredients in a food processor or high-powered blender, and serve.

Veggie Fajitas Tacos

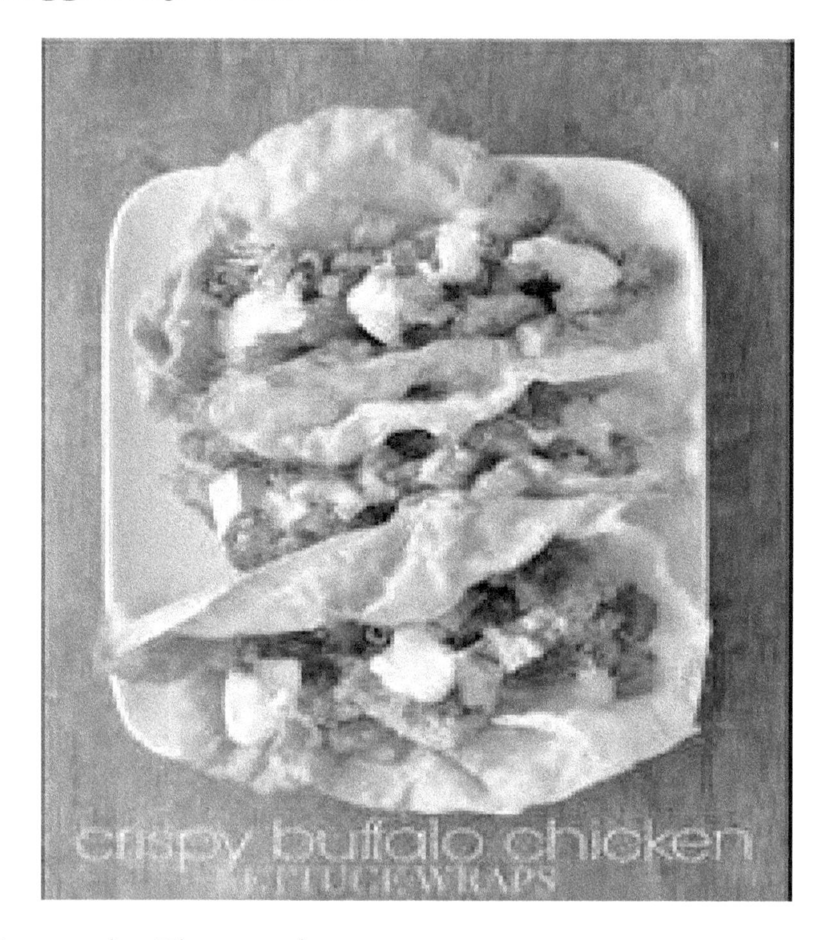

Preparation Time: 5 minutes

Cooking Time: 30 minutes

Servings: 2

Ingredients

2-3 large portobello mushrooms

2 bell peppers

1 onion

Juice of 1/2 key lime

1 tbsp grapeseed oil

6 corn-free tortillas (look for tortillas made with approved grains, like spelt or wild rice)

Your choice of approved seasonings (onion powder, habanero, cayenne pepper)

Avocado

Directions:

Remove stems of mushrooms, spoon out gills if desired, and wipe tops clean. Cut into about 1/3-inch thick slices.

Thinly slice bell peppers and onion.

In a large skillet over medium heat, add 1 Tbsp. grapeseed oil and peppers and onions. Cook about 2 minutes.

Add mushrooms and seasonings. Stir occasionally, cook another 7-8 minutes or until softened.

Warm tortillas and spoon the fajita mixture into the center of the tortillas. Serve with avocado and key lime juice.

Healthy “Fried-Rice”

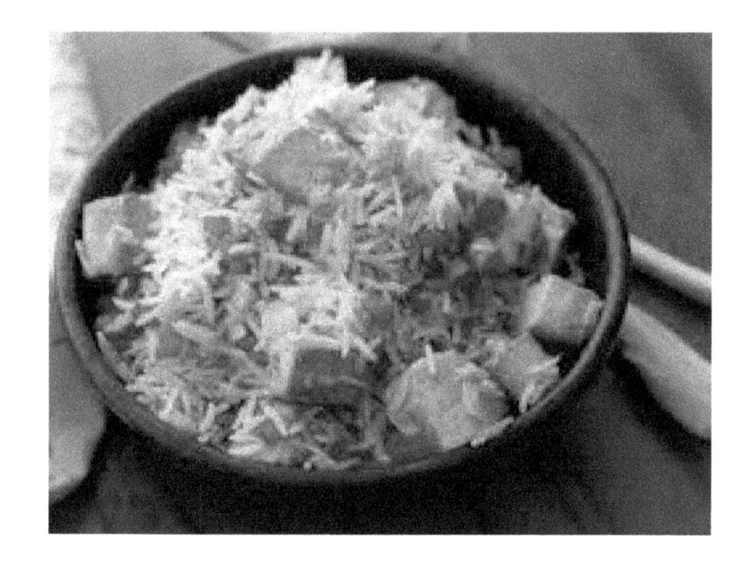

Preparation Time: 5 minutes

Cooking Time: 20 minutes

Servings: 2

Ingredients:

1 cup cooked wild rice or quinoa

1/2 cup sliced bell peppers

1/2 cup sliced mushrooms

1/2 cup sliced zucchini

1/4 onion, cubed

1 tbsp grapeseed oil

Sea salt and cayenne pepper, to taste

Directions:

Heat oil in a pan, and sautée onion until browned.

Add remaining vegetables and cook for another 5 minutes. Make sure they're not too soft.

Add the cup of boiled rice and continue cooking until lightly browned.

"Zoodles" With Avocado Sauce

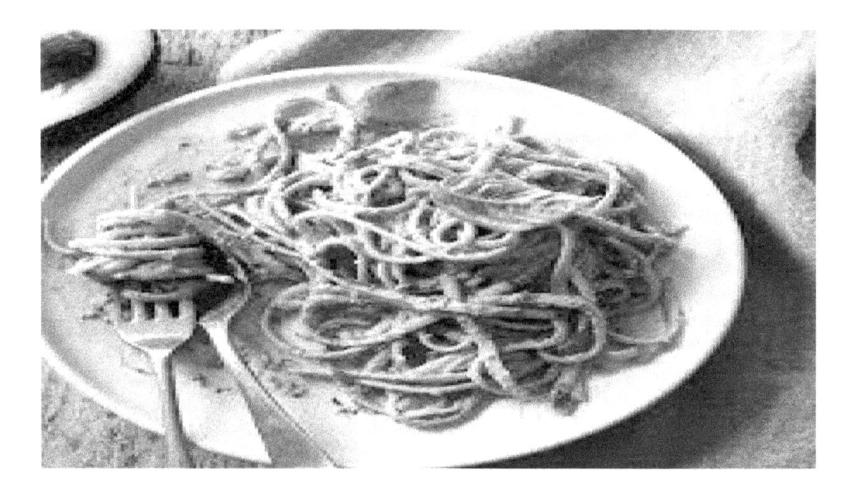

Preparation Time: 5 minutes

Cooking Time: 30 minutes

Servings: 2

Ingredients:

2 large zucchinis

2 cups basil

1/2 cup water

1/2 cup walnuts

4 tbsp key lime juice

2 avocados

24 sliced cherry tomatoes

Sea salt, to taste.

Directions:

Make zucchini noodles using a peeler or Spiralizer.

Blend the rest of the ingredients (except the cherry tomatoes) in a blender until smooth.

Combine noodles, avocado sauce and cherry tomatoes in a mixing bowl.

Garlic butter gnocchi with crispy purple sprouting broccoli

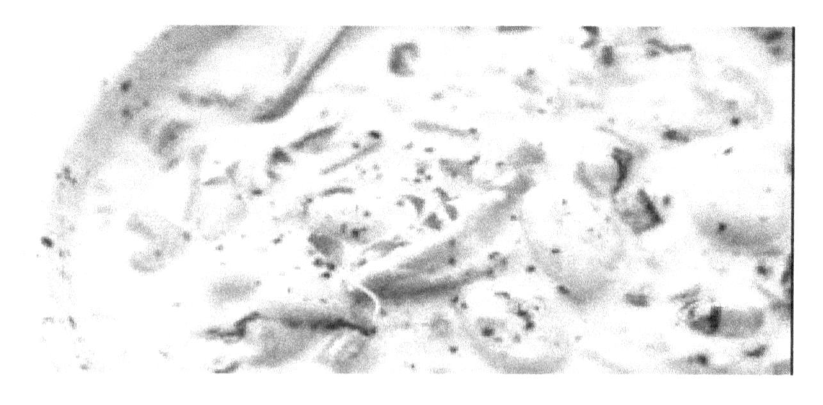

Preparation Time: 5 minutes

Cooking Time: 20 minutes

Servings: 2

Ingredients:

1 tbsp olive oil

200g purple sprouting broccoli, trimmed

500g gnocchi

½ lemon, juiced

Sauce

1 tbsp olive oil

1 onion, finely chopped

4 garlic cloves, finely chopped or crushed

1 red chili, finely chopped

75g butter

1 lemon, juiced

30g parmesan (or veggie alternative), finely grated, plus extra to serve

½ tsp Dijon mustard

Directions:

Heat the olive oil in a pan over a medium heat and fry the broccoli for 5-10 minutes or until it begins to crisp up.

While the broccoli is frying, make the sauce. Heat a medium/large frying pan over a medium heat and add the olive oil. Cook the onion until turning translucent, then add the garlic and chilli, and cook for 5 minutes. Add in the butter, lemon juice, parmesan, mustard and plenty of seasoning, and cook on a low-medium heat until the cheese is melted and everything is combined (reserve a little sauce to drizzle over the broccoli). Simmer over a low heat while you cook the gnocchi following pack instructions. Drain the gnocchi, saving a little of the cooking water, and tip everything into the sauce, adding a little of the reserved cooking water to loosen, if needed.

Serve in warm bowls topped with the broccoli, a squeeze of lemon juice and extra parmesan, if you like.

Amaranth Porridge

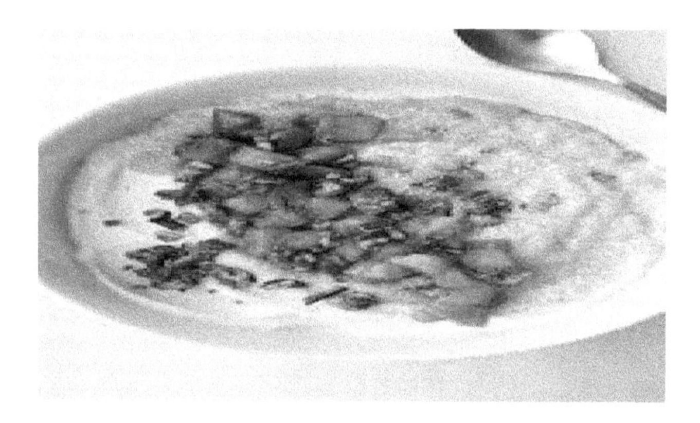

Preparation Time: 5 minutes

Cooking Time: 30 minutes

Servings: 2.

Ingredients:

2 cups coconut milk

2 cups alkaline water

1 cup amaranth

2 tbsps. coconut oil

1 tbsp. ground cinnamon

Directions:

In a saucepan, mix in the milk with water then boil the mixture.

You stir in the amaranth then reduce the heat to medium.

Cook on the medium heat then simmer for at least 30 minutes as you stir it occasionally.

Turn off the heat.

Add in cinnamon and coconut oil then stir.

Serve.

Banana Barley Porridge

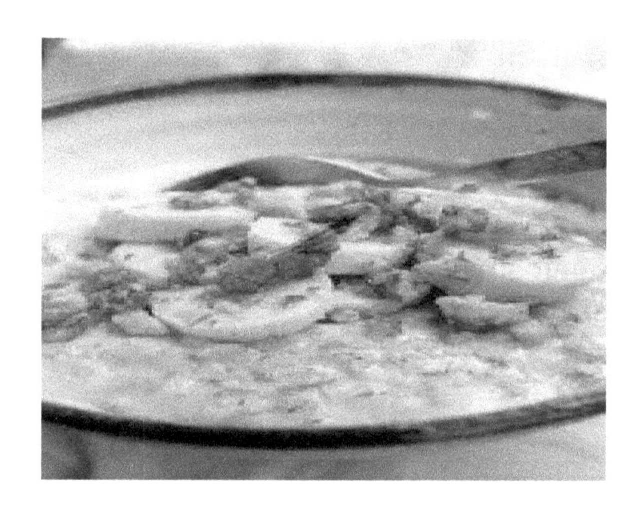

Preparation Time: 15 minutes

Cooking Time: 5 minutes

Servings: 2

Ingredients:

1 cup divided unsweetened coconut milk

1 small peeled and sliced banana

1/2 cup barley

3 drops liquid stevia

1/4 cup chopped coconuts

Directions:

In a bowl, properly mix barley with half of the coconut milk and stevia.

Cover the bowl then refrigerate for about 6 hours.

In a saucepan, mix the barley mixture with coconut milk.

Cook for about 5 minutes on moderate heat.

Then top it with the chopped coconuts and the banana slices.

Serve.

Zucchini Muffins

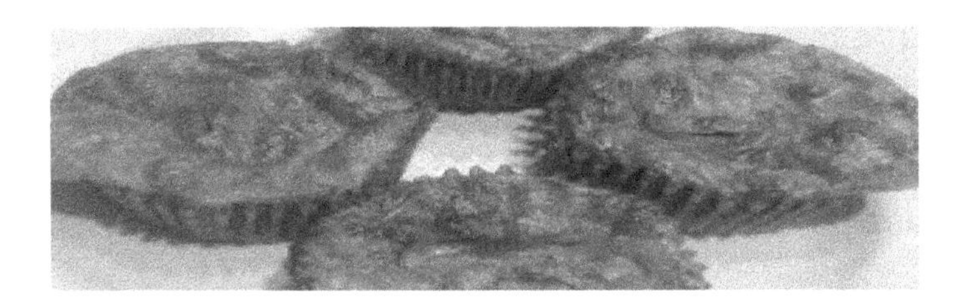

Preparation Time: 10 minutes

Cooking Time: 25 minutes

Servings: 16

Ingredients:

1 tbsp. ground flaxseed

3 tbsps. alkaline water

1/4 cup walnut butter

3 medium over-ripe bananas

2 small grated zucchinis

1/2 cup coconut milk

1 tsp. vanilla extract

2 cups coconut flour

1 tbsp. baking powder

1 tsp. cinnamon

1/4 tsp. sea salt

Directions:

Adjust the temperature of your oven to 375°F.

Grease the muffin tray with the cooking spray.

In a bowl, mix the flaxseed with water.

In a glass bowl, mash the bananas then stir in the remaining ingredients.

Properly mix and then divide the mixture into the muffin tray.

Bake it for 25 minutes.

Serve.

Millet Porridge

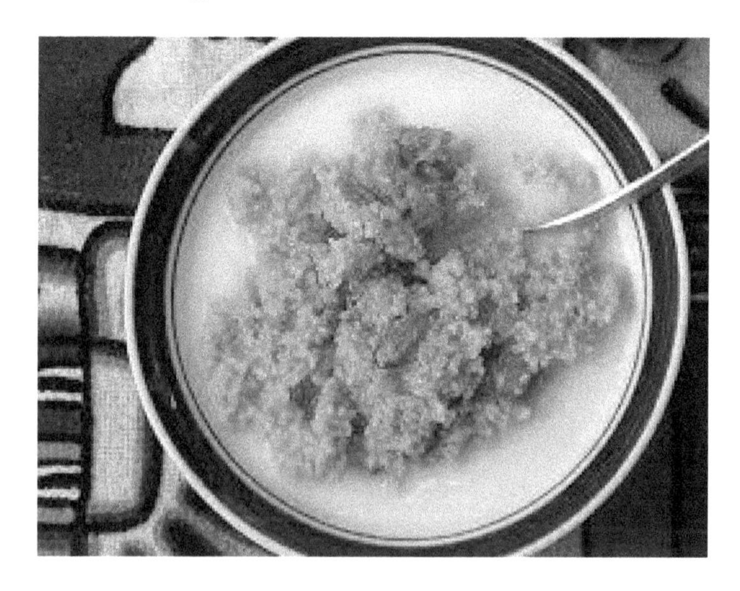

Preparation Time: 10 minutes

Cooking Time: 20 minutes

Servings: 2

Ingredients:

Sea salt

1 tbsp. finely chopped coconuts

1/2 cup unsweetened coconut milk

1/2 cup rinsed and drained millet

1-1/2 cups alkaline water

3 drops liquid stevia

Directions:

Sauté the millet in a non-stick skillet for about 3 minutes.

Add salt and water then stir.

Let the meal boil then reduce the amount of heat.

Cook for about 15 minutes then add the remaining ingredients. Stir.

Cook the meal for 4 extra minutes.

Serve the meal with toping of the chopped nuts.

Jackfruit Vegetable Fry

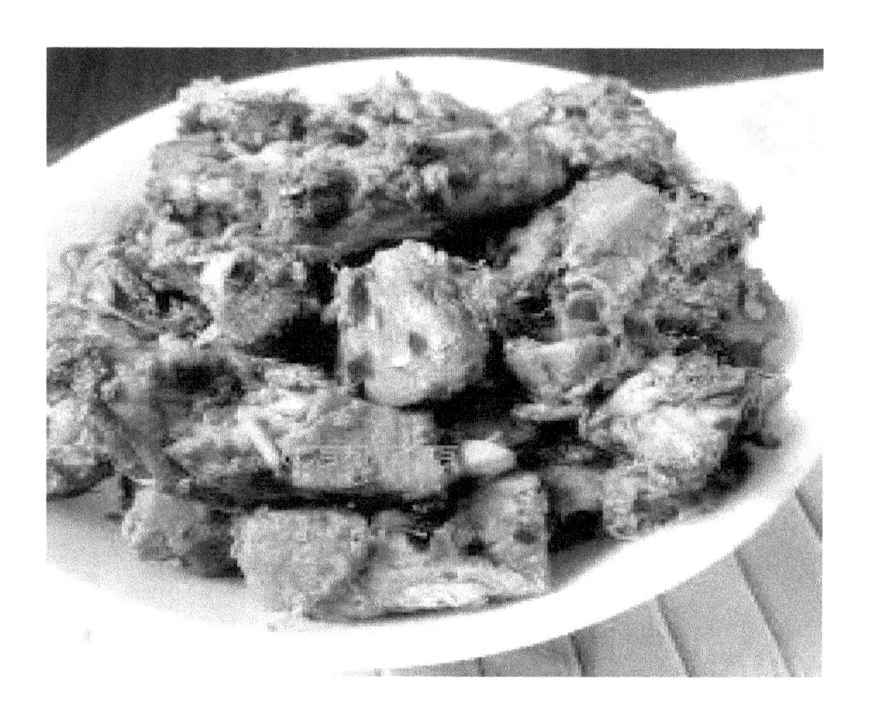

Preparation Time: 5 minutes

Cooking Time: 5 minutes

Servings: 6

Ingredients:

2 finely chopped small onions

2 cups finely chopped cherry tomatoes

1/8 tsp. ground turmeric

1 tbsp. olive oil

2 seeded and chopped red bell peppers

3 cups seeded and chopped firm jackfruit

1/8 tsp. cayenne pepper

2 tbsps. chopped fresh basil leaves

Salt

Directions:

In a greased skillet, sauté the onions and bell peppers for about 5 minutes.

Add the tomatoes then stir.

Cook for 2 minutes.

Then add the jackfruit, cayenne pepper, salt, and turmeric.

Cook for about 8 minutes.

Garnish the meal with basil leaves.

Serve warm.

Zucchini Pancakes

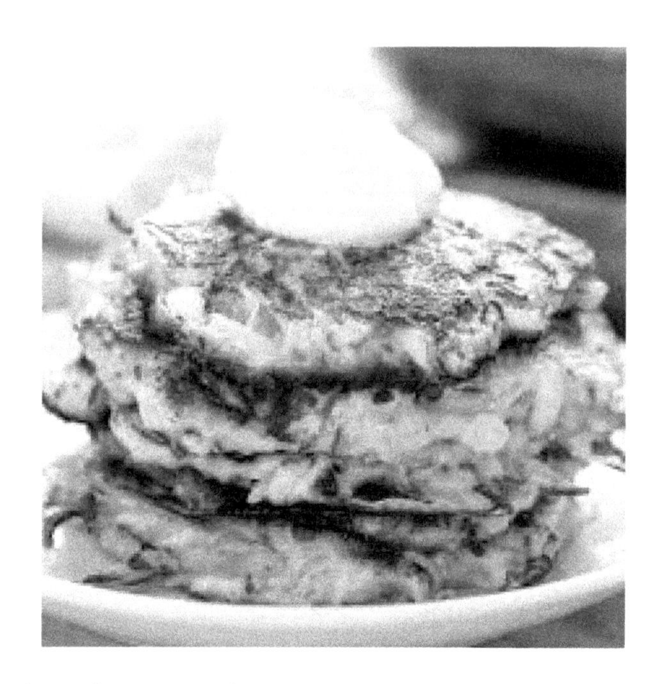

Preparation Time: 15 minutes

Cooking Time: 8 minutes

Servings: 8

Ingredients:

12 tbsps. alkaline water

6 large grated zucchinis

Sea salt

4 tbsps. ground Flax Seeds

2 tsps. olive oil

2 finely chopped jalapeño peppers

1/2 cup finely chopped scallions

Directions:

In a bowl, mix together water and the flax seeds then set it aside.

Pour oil in a large non-stick skillet then heat it on medium heat.

Then add the black pepper, salt, and zucchini.

Cook for 3 minutes then transfer the zucchini into a large bowl.

Add the flaxseed and the scallion's mixture then properly mix it.

Preheat a griddle then grease it lightly with the cooking spray.

Pour 1/4 of the zucchini mixture into griddle then cook for 3 minutes.

Flip the side carefully then cook for 2 more minutes.

Repeat the procedure with the remaining mixture in batches.

Serve.

Squash Hash

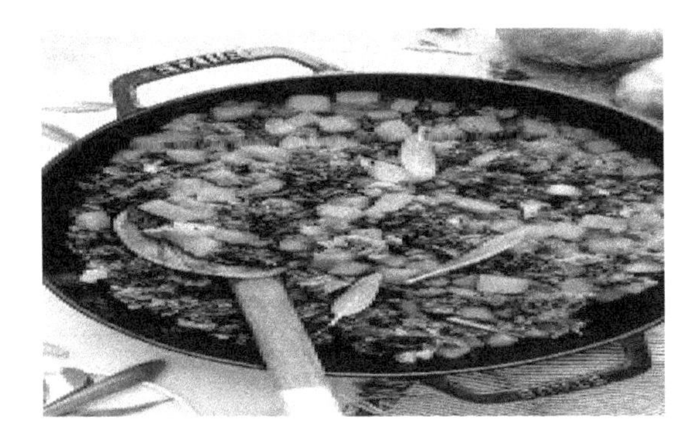

Preparation Time: 2 minutes

Cooking Time: 10 minutes

Servings: 2

Ingredients:

1 tsp. onion powder

1/2 cup finely chopped onion

2 cups spaghetti squash

1/2 tsp. sea salt

Directions:

Using paper towels, squeeze extra moisture from spaghetti squash.

Place the squash into a bowl then add the salt, onion, and the onion powder.

Stir properly to mix them.

Spray a non-stick cooking skillet with cooking spray then place it over moderate heat.

Add the spaghetti squash to pan.

Cook the squash for about 5 minutes.

Flip the hash browns using a spatula.

Cook for an extra 5 minutes until the desired crispness is reached.

Serve.

Hemp Seed Porridge

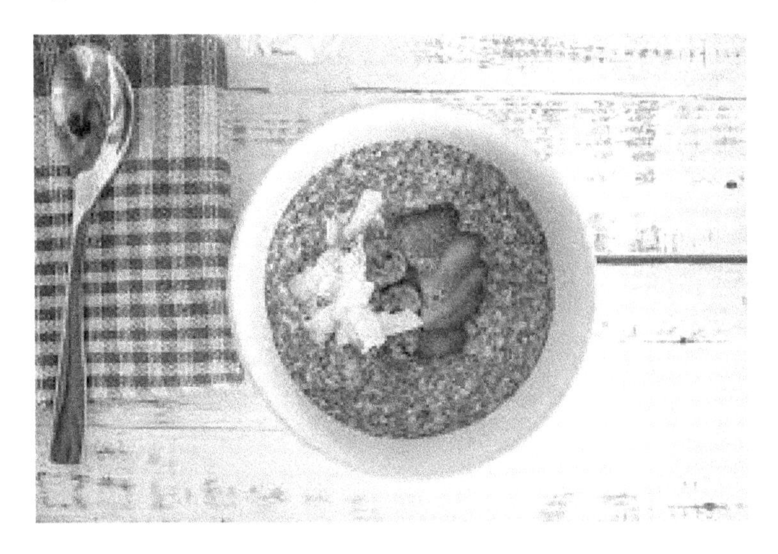

Preparation Time: 5 minutes

Cooking Time: 5 minutes

Servings: 6

Ingredients:

3 cups cooked hemp seed

1 packet Stevia

1 cup coconut milk

Directions:

In a saucepan, mix the rice and the coconut milk over moderate heat for about 5 minutes as you stir it constantly.

Remove the pan from the heat then add the Stevia. Stir.

Serve in 6 bowls.

Enjoy.

Main dishes

Cauliflower Potato Curry

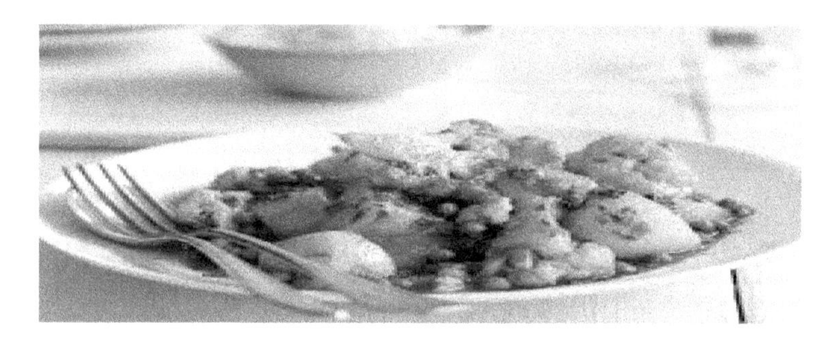

Preparation Time: 10 minutes

Cooking Time: 35 minutes

Servings: 4

Ingredients:

2 tbsps. vegetable oil

1 large chopped onion

A large grated piece of ginger

3 finely chopped chive stalks

1/2 tsp. turmeric

1 tsp. ground cumin

1 tsp. curry powder

1 cup chopped tomatoes

1/2 tsp. sugar

1 florets cauliflower

2 chopped potatoes

1 small halved lengthways green chili

A squeeze seville orange juice

Handful roughly chopped coriander

Directions:

Add the onion to a greased skillet then sauté until soft.

Add all the spices in the skillet then stir.

Add the cauliflower and potatoes.

Sauté for about 5 minutes then add green chilies tomatoes, and sugar.

Cover then cook for about 30 minutes.

Serve warm with the coriander and seville orange juice.

Vegetable Bean Curry

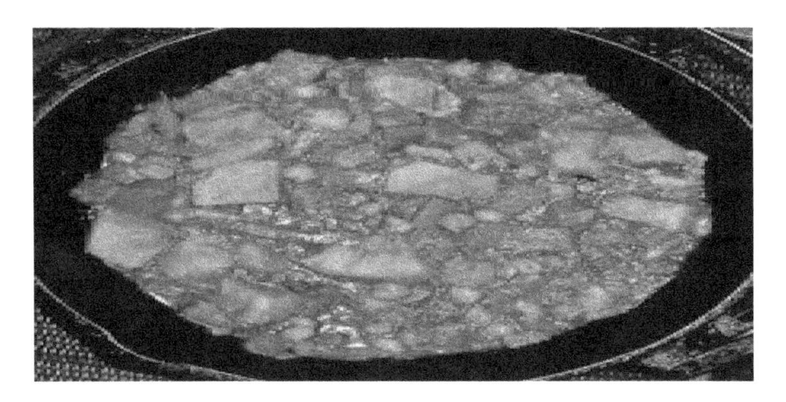

Preparation Time: 5 minutes

Cooking Time: 6 hours

Servings: 8

Ingredients:

1 finely chopped onion

4 chopped chive stalks

3 tsps. coriander powder

1/2 tsp. cinnamon powder

1 tsp. ginger powder

1 tsp. turmeric powder

1/2 tsp. cayenne pepper

2 tbsps. tomato paste

1 tbsp. avocado oil

2 cans,15 ounces each, rinsed and drained lima beans

3 cups cubed and peeled turnips

3 cups fresh cauliflower florets

4 medium diced zucchinis

2 medium seeded and chopped tomatoes

2 cups vegetable broth

1 cup light coconut milk

1/2 tsp. pepper

1/4 tsp. sea salt

Directions:

In a slow cooker, preheat the oil then add all the vegetables.

Add in the remaining ingredients then stir.

Cook for about 6 hours at low temperature.

Serve warm.

Wild Mushroom Soup

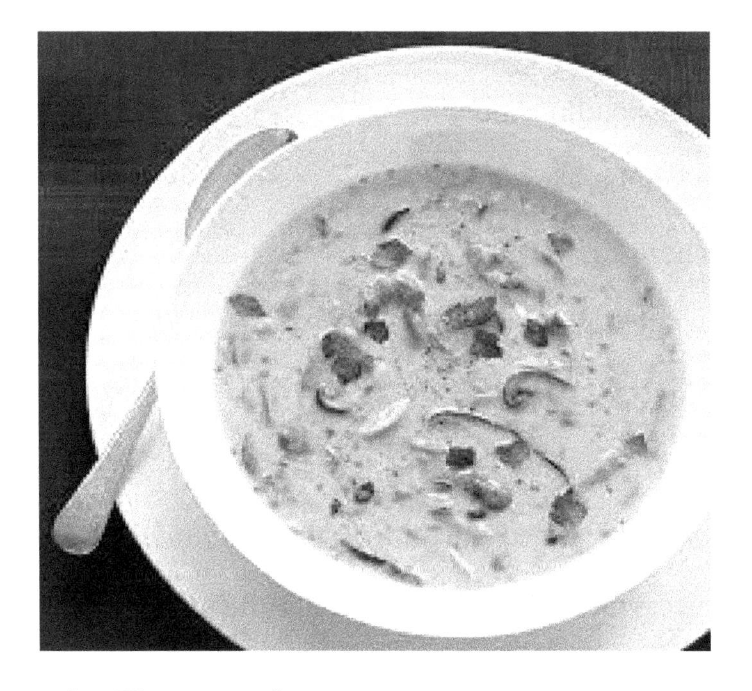

Preparation Time: 10 minutes

Cooking Time: 15 minutes

Servings: 4

Ingredients:

4 oz. walnut butter

1 chopped shallot

5 oz. chopped portabella mushrooms

5 oz. chopped oyster mushrooms

5 oz. chopped shiitake mushrooms

1 minced chive clove

1/2 tsp. dried thyme

3 cups alkaline water

1 vegetable bouillon cube

1 cup coconut cream

1/2 lb. chopped celery root

1 tbsp. white wine vinegar

Fresh cilantro

Directions:

In a cooking pan, melt the butter over medium heat.

Add the vegetables into the pan then sauté until golden brown.

Add the remaining ingredients to the pan then properly mix it.

Boil the mixture.

Simmer it for 15 minutes on low heat.

Add the cream to the soup then pour it using a handheld blender.

Serve warm with the chopped cilantro as toppings.

Grilled Vegetable Stack

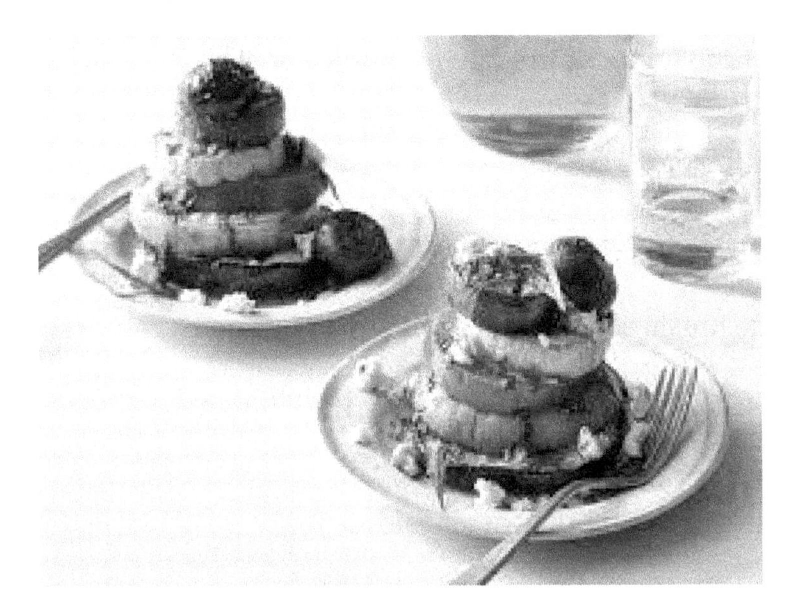

Preparation Time: 10 minutes

Cooking Time: 20 minutes

Servings: 2

Ingredients:

1/2 zucchini, sliced into slices about 1/4-inch thick

2 stemmed Portobello mushrooms with the gills removed

1 tsp. divided sea salt

1/2 cup divided hummus

1 peeled and sliced red onion

1 seeded red bell pepper, sliced lengthwise

1 seeded yellow bell pepper, sliced lengthwise

Directions:

Adjust the temperature of your broiler or grill.

Grill the mushroom caps over coal or gas flame.

Add the yellow and red bell peppers, onion, and zucchini for about 20 minutes as you turn it occasionally.

Fill the mushroom cap with 1/4 cup of hummus.

Top it with some onion, yellow peppers, red peppers, and zucchini.

Add salt to season then set it aside.

Repeat the process with the second mushroom cap and the remaining ingredients.

Serve.

Bok Choy Soup

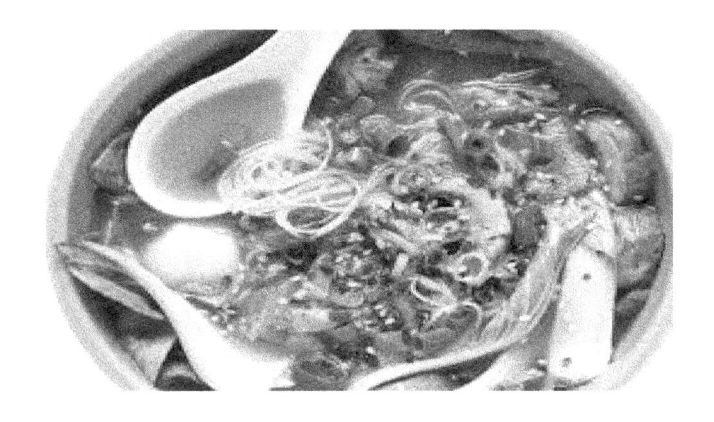

Preparation Time: 5 minutes

Cooking Time: 10 minutes

Servings: 2

Ingredients:

1 cup chopped Bok Choy

3 cups vegetable broth

2 peeled and sliced zucchinis

1/2 cup cooked hemp seed

1 roughly chopped bunch radish

Directions:

In a pan, mix the ingredients over moderate heat.

Let it simmer then cook it for about 10 minutes until the vegetables become tender.

Serve.

Mushroom Cheese Steak

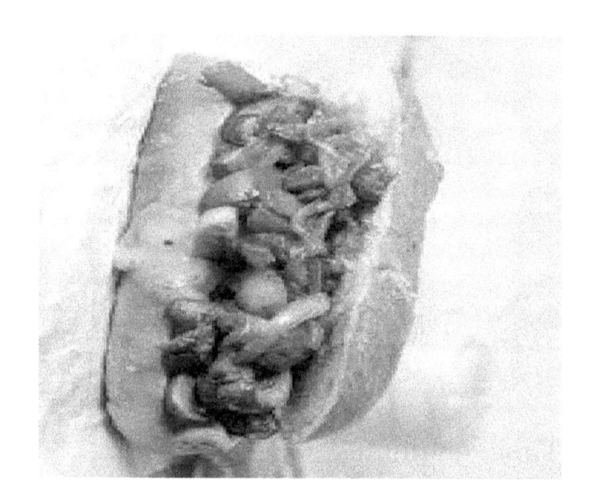

Preparation Time: 5 minutes

Cooking Time: 20 minutes

Servings: 2

Mushrooms:

Savory, 1 tsp.

Grapeseed oil, 1 tbsp

Red bell pepper, 1 c

Thyme, 1 tsp.

Green bell pepper, 1 c

Oregano, 1 tsp.

Sliced onion, 1 c

Smoked sea salt, 1 tsp.

Portabella mushroom caps, 4

Onion powder, 1 tbsp

Cheese:

Basil, .5 tsp.

Sea salt, .5 tsp.

Cayenne, .5 tsp.

Hemp seeds, 1.5 tsp.

Springwater, .33 to .5 c

Oregano, .5 tsp.

Soaked brazil nuts, .75 c

Onion powder, 1.5 tsp.

Directions:

Take the mushrooms and slice them very thinly.

Beat all of the seasonings together with just enough olive oil to make a marinade.

Add the mushrooms into the marinade and let them rest for 30 minutes. Stir them halfway through.

As those marinate, add all of the ingredients for the cheese into a blender. Turn the blender on until all ingredients are smooth.

Pour the grapeseed oil into a skillet and add the peppers and onions. Sauté them for three to five minutes. Mix in the mushrooms and sauté for another five minutes. Serve topped with the cheese.

Enjoy as-is, or on a flatbread.

Squash Falafels

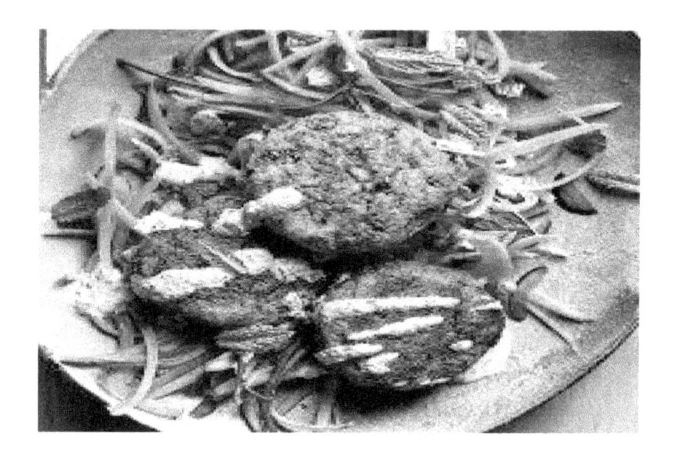

Preparation Time: 5 minutes

Cooking Time: 20 minutes

Servings: 2

Ingredients:

Grapeseed oil, 1 tbsp

Sea salt

Chickpea flour, .5 c

Cayenne pepper, 1 tbsp

Small white onion

Dried oregano, 2 tbsp

Fresh coriander, 3 tbsp

Fresh parsley, 3 tbsp

Tahini, 1 tbsp

Cooked chickpeas, 3 c

Dried dill, 2 tbsp

Butternut squash, 1c

Onion powder, 2 tbsp

Dressing:

Water, .25 c

Tahini, 2 tbsp

Dried dill, 1 tsp.

Juice of a lime

Dried oregano, 1 tsp.

Sea salt

Cayenne pepper, .5 tsp.

Directions:

Start out by steaming your butternut squash for at least 20 minutes. You can check for softness by piercing a piece with a fork. If the fork goes in easily, it is done.

Once the butternut squash is prepared, add the squash, chickpeas, tahini, parsley, coriander, onion powder, dill, oregano, cayenne, onion, chickpea flour, salt, and grapeseed oil to a food processor. Mix it all together until it forms a moist dough.

Using an ice cream scooper, scoop out the falafel mixture on a parchment-lined cookie sheet. Once you have scooped out all of the dough, all the falafels to bake for 20 minutes and 400.

As the falafels cook, add all of the dressing recipes to a bowl and mix together using a whisk or fork. You can adjust the amount of water depending on how thin you want it to be.

Once everything is done, you can serve the falafels on homemade flatbread along with a drizzle of the dressing. Enjoy.

Home Fries

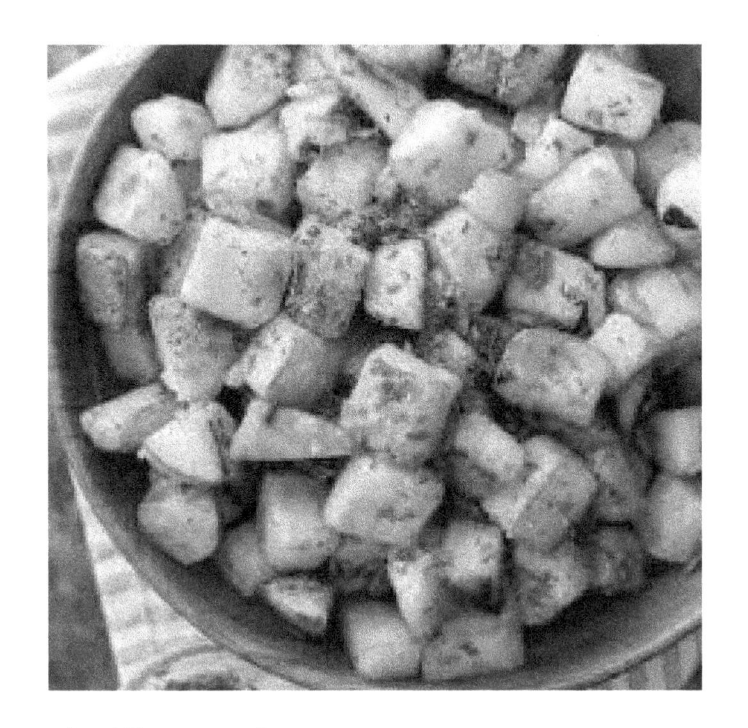

Preparation Time: 5 minutes

Cooking Time: 25 minutes

Servings: 2

Ingredients:

Grapeseed oil

Cayenne pepper, .5 tsp.

Diced plum tomato

Oregano, 1 tsp.

Diced green bell pepper, .25 c

Sea salt, 1 tsp.

Diced onion, .25 c

Green bananas, 3

Directions:

To get the best results with this recipe, make sure that your bananas still have green skin. Green skinned bananas should be firm, and they tend to taste a lot like potatoes when they are cooked. The more yellow the skin is, the more it will taste like banana and the softer they will become when cooked.

Begin by chopping the end off of each of the bananas and then slice them in half. Then slice each of the halves lengthwise. Carefully wedge your finger between the banana and the skin and pull the skin off.

Slice the bananas thinly and then place it in a bowl. Pour the oil over them and gently toss them to coat. Add all of the seasonings and toss them all together. Let this rest for about five to ten minutes.

Add about two tablespoons of oil into a large skillet and let it heat up to medium. Add in the home fries. Keep them spread evenly across the pan. Add in the tomatoes, peppers, and onions.

Continue to cook everything for five to seven minutes before you start flipping the food. Flip them, and then let them cook for another five minutes, stirring occasionally.

You can enjoy these as they are or with some alkaline ketchup.

Chicken Tenders

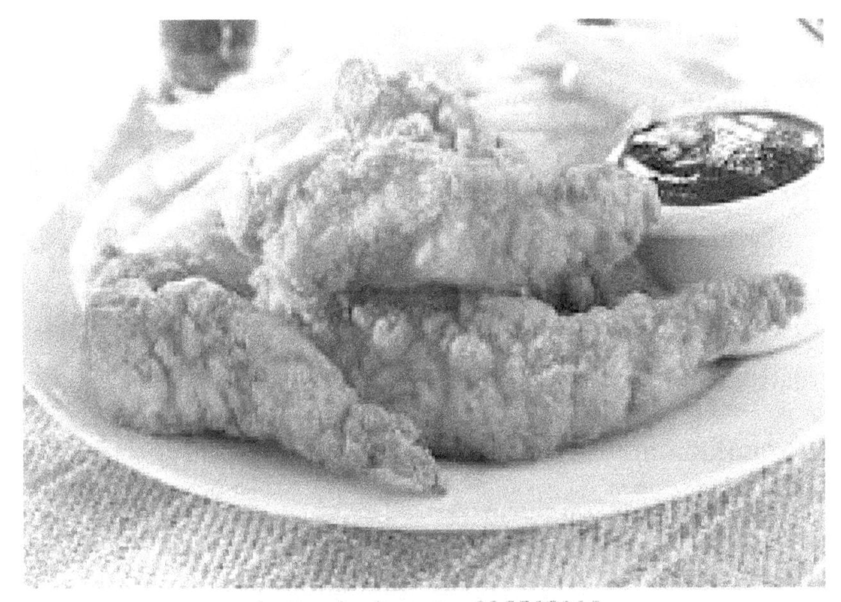

Preparation Time: 5 minutes

Cooking Time: 30 minutes

Servings: 2

Ingredients:

Sage, 2 tsp.

Grapeseed oil

Allspice, 1 tsp.

Sea salt, 2 tsp.

Basil, 2 tsp.

Oregano, 2 tsp.

Spelt Flour, 1.5 c

Cayenne pepper, 1 tsp.

Aquafaba or Springwater, 1.5 c

Ginger powder, 2 tsp.

Portabella mushrooms, 2 to 6

Onion powder, 2 tsp.

Directions:

The aquafaba mentioned above is simply the water that comes off of garbanzo beans.

To start, slice the mushroom caps into half-inch slices and then lay them in a large bowl. You can use the mushroom stems to make "chicken" nuggets. Add half of each of the seasonings, aquafaba, and some of the oil into the container and mix everything together so that the mushrooms are coated. Let this sit and marinate for about an hour. Mix together the remaining seasonings and the flour together. Coat all of the mushroom pieces in the flour mixture.

Make sure that you have your oven to 400. Brush some oil on a baking sheet a lay the mushroom pieces across the baking sheet. Allow them to bake for 15 minutes, flip them over, and then let them cook for another 15 minutes, or until they are crispy. Enjoy them as is, or place them on some Dr. Sebi approved bread.

Veggies with Mushrooms

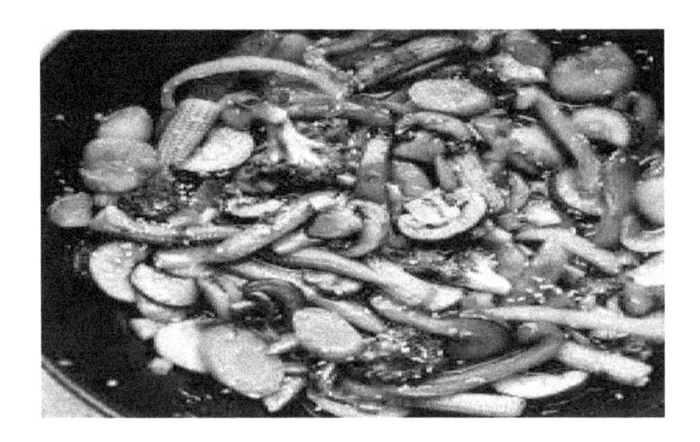

Preparation Time: 5 minutes

Cooking Time: 10 minutes

Servings: 4

Ingredients:

1 tsp. coconut oil

1 cup sliced mushroom

1/2 cup chopped onion

2 tbsps. smashed chive

2 tbsps. finely chopped ginger

1-1/2 tbsps. sambal Oelek

1-1/2 cups chopped cabbage

2 cups chopped leeks, white part only

1/2 cup chopped celery

2 tbsps. sliced jalapenos

1/4 cup sliced green bell peppers

3 tbsps. vegetable stock

Directions:

In a greased skillet sauté the onion and mushrooms for about 3 minutes.

Stir in the chive, ginger, Sambal Oelek then sauté for 30 seconds.

Add in the leeks, cabbage, peppers then cook for about 2 minutes.

Add the pepper and salt to season.

Add the vegetable stock then cook for 1 minute.

Serve warm.

Rosemary Roasted Yams

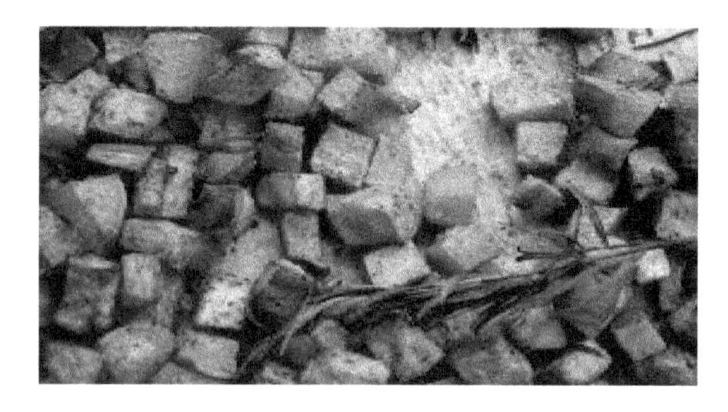

Preparation Time: 10 minutes

Cooking Time: 45 minutes

Servings: 4

Ingredients:

2 cups cubed yams

1 tbsp. coconut oil

6 fresh rosemary sprigs leave with removed and finely chopped stems discarded

Iodine free Celtic sea salt

Black pepper

Directions:

Adjust the temperature of the oven to 375°F.

In a bowl, mix in the yams with oil and rosemary.

Spread the yams on a baking sheet.

Bake for about 50 minutes.

Add salt and pepper to season.

Serve warm.

Soy-And-Butter-Braised Mushrooms

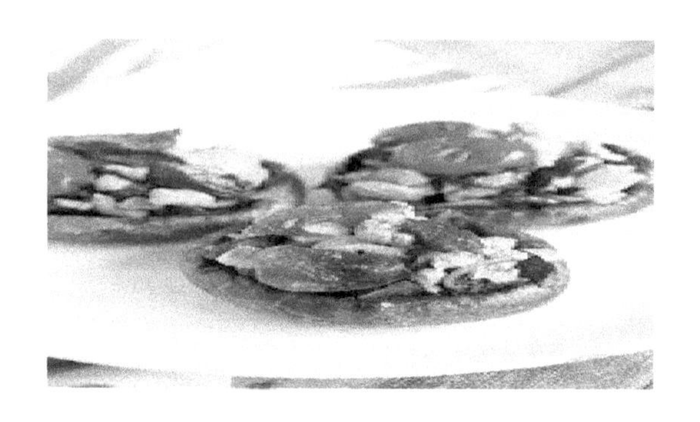

Preparation Time: 5 minutes

Cooking Time: 20 minutes

Servings: 2

Ingredients:

50g butter

6 medium flat mushrooms

6 spring onions, chopped, plus extra to serve

a thumb-sized piece of ginger, chopped

1 red chili, finely chopped

3 tbsp soy sauce

a pinch of caster sugar

150g basmati rice

2 tsp toasted sesame oil

Directions:

Heat the butter in a large frying pan. Fry the mushrooms for 3-4 minutes, turning as they cook. Add 1/2 the spring onions and all the ginger, chili, soy sauce and sugar. Keep turning the mushrooms in the sauce until they are cooked and the sauce is glossy but still liquid. Cook the basmati following pack instructions then stir through the rest of the spring onions and the sesame oil. Spoon the rice into bowls, add the mushrooms and spoon over the sauce. Finish with a few more chopped spring onions, if you like.

Super-Seedy Salad with Tahini Dressing

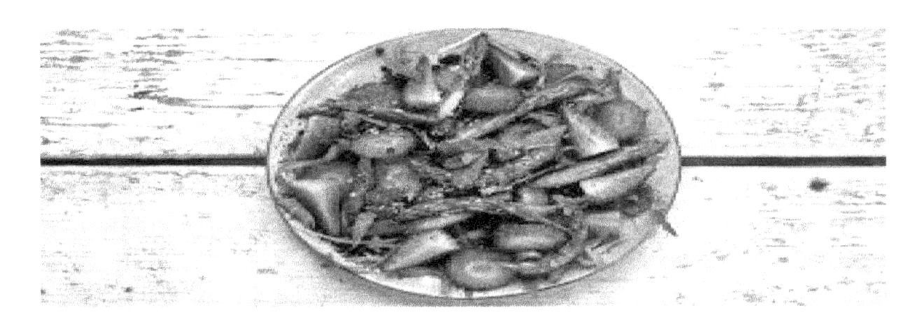

Preparation Time: 5 minutes

Cooking Time: 30 minutes

Servings: 2

Ingredients:

1 slice stale sourdough, torn into chunks

50g mixed seeds

1 tsp cumin seeds

1 tsp coriander seeds

a good pinch of dried chili flakes

spray oil

50g baby kale

75g long-stemmed broccoli, blanched for a few minutes then roughly chopped

½ red onion, thinly sliced

100g cherry tomatoes, halved

½ a small bunch flat-leaf parsley, torn

Dressing

100ml natural yogurt

1 tbsp tahini

1 lemon, juiced

Directions:

Heat the oven to 200°C/fan 180°C/gas 6. Put the bread into a food processor and pulse into very rough breadcrumbs. Put into a bowl with the mixed seeds and spices, season, and spray well with oil. Tip onto a nonstick baking tray and roast for 15-20 minutes, stirring and tossing regularly, until deep golden brown. Cool.

Whisk together the dressing ingredients, some seasoning and a splash of water in a large bowl. Tip the baby kale, broccoli, red onion, cherry tomatoes and flat leaf parsley into the dressing, and mix well. Divide between 2 plates and top with the crispy breadcrumbs and seeds.

Rice-Stuffed Omelette With Pickled Cucumber

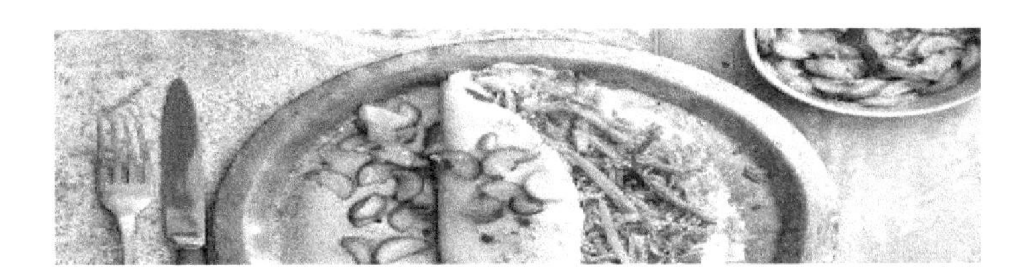

Preparation Time: 5 minutes

Cooking Time: 30 minutes

Servings: 2

Ingredients:

vegetable or groundnut oil for frying

4 spring onions, shredded

1 carrot, shredded

250g pouch cooked basmati rice

1 tbsp soy sauce

2 tsp ginger, finely grated

6 eggs, beaten

1 tbsp mirin

sesame oil

sesame seeds, toasted, to serve

Pickled Cucumber

2 mini cucumbers, halved lengthways and sliced

1 tbsp rice vinegar

1 tsp caster sugar

a pinch of dried chili flakes

Directions:

Put the cucumbers in a bowl with the vinegar, sugar, chili flakes, and a pinch of salt. Toss and leave while you cook the omelette.

Heat a little vegetable oil in a pan then fry the vegetables for a few minutes until soft. Tip in the rice and stir, then add the soy sauce, 1/2 the ginger and stir-fry until hot.

Beat the eggs with the mirin, the remaining ginger and a few drops of sesame oil.

Heat more vegetable oil in a small, non-stick frying pan then pour in 1/2 the beaten eggs. Cook gently until the base is set but the top is still moist. Put on a warmed plate and make another omelette with the rest of the egg.

Spoon the rice mixture over each omelette, fold and serve with the pickled cucumber and a scattering of sesame seeds, if you like.

Baked feta with lentils, chilli and herbs

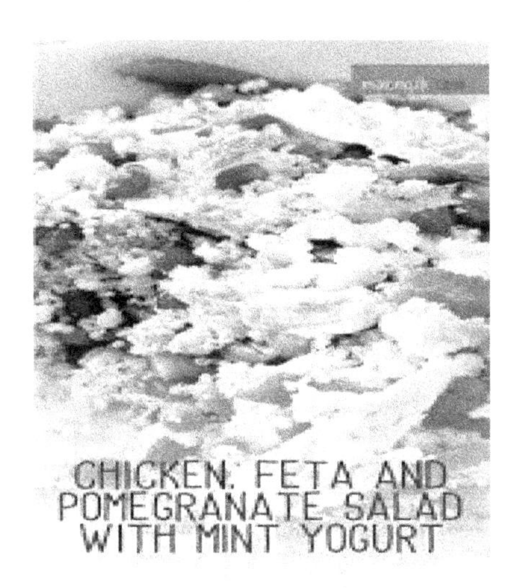

Preparation Time: 5 minutes

Cooking Time: 40 minutes

Servings: 2

Ingredients:

200g block feta

½ red onion, finely sliced

1 red chili, finely chopped

2 tbsp olive oil

1 lemon, halved

250g pack of ready-to-eat puy lentils

handful of mint, chopped

handful of coriander, chopped

crusty bread, to serve

Directions:

Heat the oven to 200°C/fan 180°C/gas 6. Cut the feta in 1/2 and sit each block on a piece of foil.

Divide the onion and chilli between the two parcels, drizzle both with 1 tbsp of olive oil and a squeeze of lemon juice, then season well and pull up the sides to make a foil boat. Bake for 15-20 minutes until it has softened or start to turn golden on the edges.

Heat the lentils following the pack instructions. Season and stir in most of the herbs then divide between two plates. Sit the feta on top and spoon over the juices from the parcels. Top with the rest of the herbs and another squeeze of lemon, and serve with crusty bread.

Courgetti with pesto and balsamic tomatoes

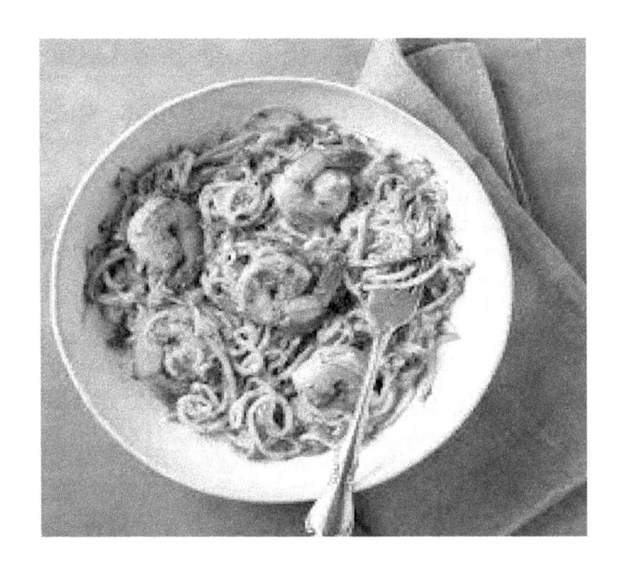

Preparation Time: 5 minutes

Cooking Time: 40 minutes

Servings: 2

Ingredients:

8 baby plum tomatoes, 4 halved and 4 whole

olive oil

1/2 clove garlic, crushed

1 tbsp balsamic vinegar

1 large courgette, spiralised or very thinly shredded into noodles

2 tbsp fresh vegetarian pesto

1 tbsp pine nuts, toasted

Directions:

Toss the tomatoes with 1 tsp oil, garlic and balsamic vinegar and some seasoning. Tip into a frying pan and cook for 5 minutes until the whole tomatoes start to burst and they are coated in the balsamic.

Pour a kettle of hot water over the courgette spaghetti and blanch for 30 seconds. Drain really well, toss with the pesto and season well. Stir, coating the noodles, then add the tomatoes and toasted pine nuts to serve your courgetti.

Buddha Bowls With Shredded Sprouts And Beets

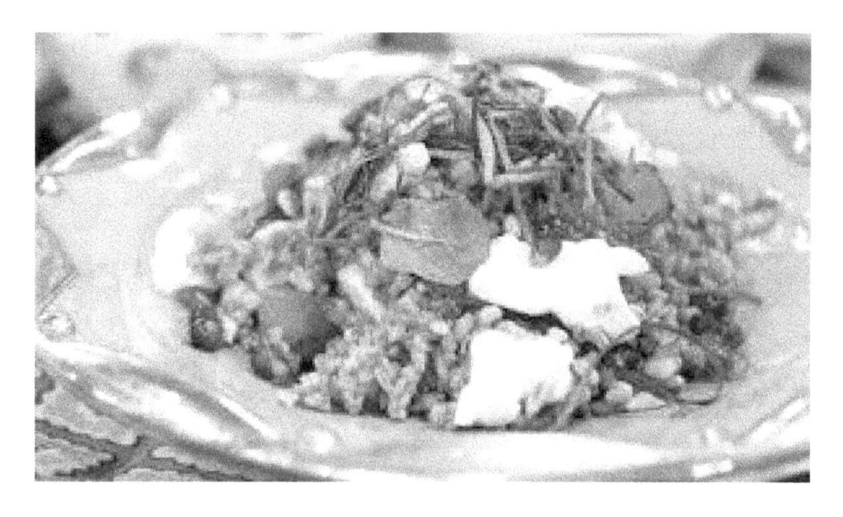

Preparation Time: 5 minutes

Cooking Time: 30 minutes

Servings: 2

Ingredients:

olive oil

1 lemon, zested and juiced

1 tbsp Dijon or wholegrain mustard

400g cooked quinoa or couscous

a handful of each, coriander and mint, chopped

2 carrots, peeled and shredded

400g tin pinto, borlotti beans or chickpeas, rinsed and drained

12 Brussels sprouts, trimmed and finely sliced

2 cooked beetroot, cubed

2 red peppers, seeded and diced

2 tbsp sunflower or pumpkin seeds, toasted

Directions:

Whisk 1 tbsp oil, lemon zest and juice, mustard and season well. Toss half the dressing with the cooked quinoa and the chopped herbs. Divide between four bowls. Top with the carrot, beans, sprouts, beetroot and pepper in piles on top of the quinoa. Spoon over the remaining dressing and scatter with the seeds to serve.

California scramble

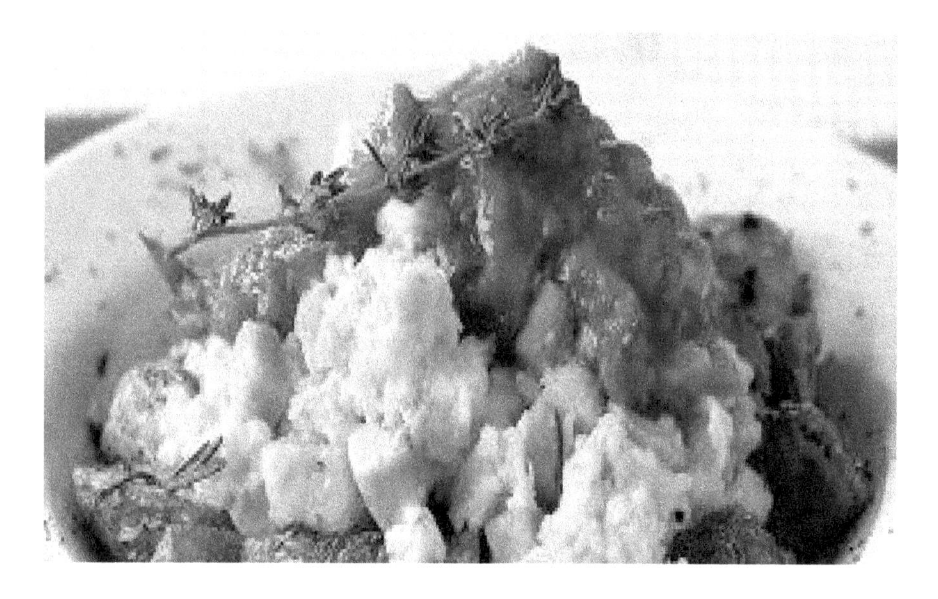

Preparation Time: 5 minutes

Cooking Time: 20 minutes

Servings: 2

Ingredients

olive oil

1 red chili, finely chopped

3 spring onions, chopped

2-3 handfuls of watercress leaves, chopped (discard the woody stalks)

3 small eggs, beaten

6 baby plum tomatoes, halved

½ small avocado, sliced

Instructions

Heat 1 tbsp of oil in a non-stick frying pan. Cook the chili and spring onion for a couple of minutes until softened then stir in half the watercress until it starts to wilt. Add the eggs and some seasoning and softly scramble.

Tip onto a warm plate and top with the rest of the watercress, tomatoes and avocado.

Pappardelle with buttery tomato and shallot sauce

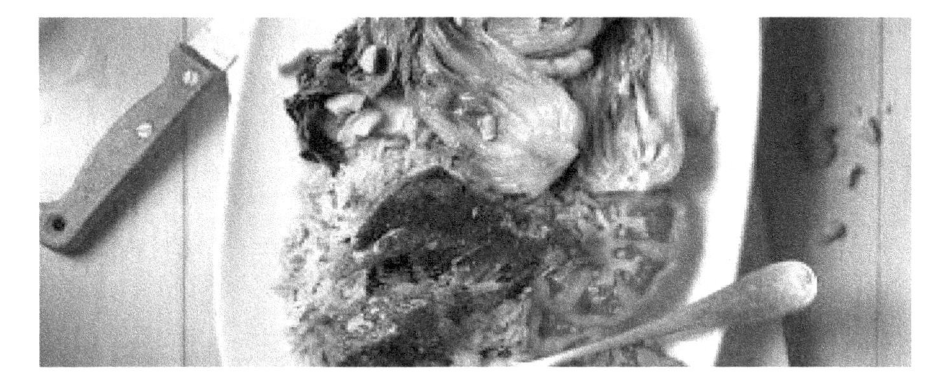

Preparation Time: 5 minutes

Cooking Time: 20 minutes

Servings: 2

Ingredients:

2 small shallots, finely sliced

50g butter

400g tin cherry tomatoes

a small bunch of basil, chopped

200g pappardelle

Directions:

Gently cook the shallots in the butter until very soft, about 5-7 minutes. Tip in the tomatoes and simmer for 10 minutes. Stir in the basil and season.

Cook the pappardelle then drain, keeping a cup of the water. Toss the pasta with the sauce, adding a little splash of pasta water to the sauce if you need to. Serve in warm bowls.

Spiced paneer with chilli green lentils

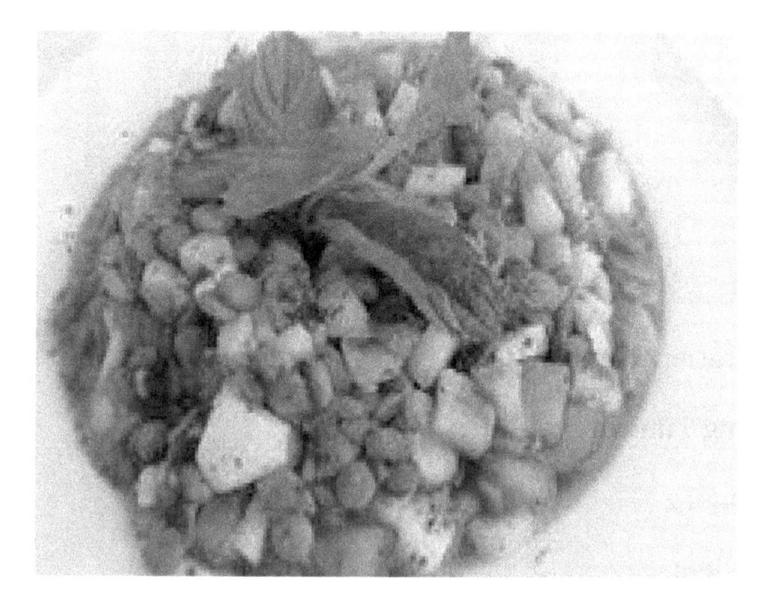

Preparation Time: 5 minutes

Cooking Time: 40 minutes

Servings: 2

Ingredients

75g green lentils

500ml vegetable stock

1 small onion, grated

a thumb-sized piece of ginger, peeled and chopped

1 red chili, finely chopped

½ tsp turmeric, plus a pinch extra

1 tsp garam masala, plus extra for the paneer

a small bunch of coriander, chopped

230g block paneer, cut into wedges or cubes

groundnut or sunflower oil

naan bread, to serve

Directions:

Put the first 7 ingredients in a pan and bring to a simmer, then cover and cook for 20 minutes, or until the lentils are tender. Drain or boil off any excess liquid, then stir in most of the coriander.

Toss the paneer with some oil, seasoning and a little more turmeric and garam masala and fry in a non-stick frying pan until golden. Spoon the lentils onto plates, top with the paneer and remaining coriander and serve with naan bread.

Coconut and peanut aubergine curry

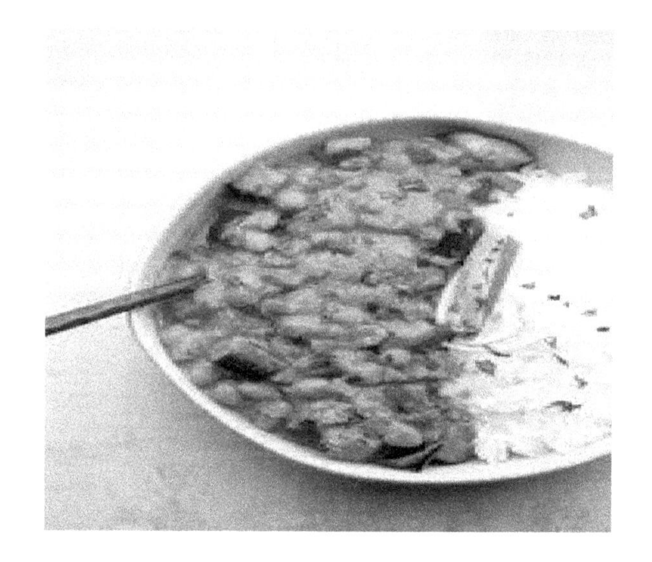

Preparation Time: 5 minutes

Cooking Time: 20 minutes

Servings: 2

Ingredients:

oil for frying

2 aubergines, cut into large chunks

2 onions, chopped

2 garlic cloves, crushed

ginger, a 5cm piece, finely grated

1 tsp cumin seeds

1 tsp coriander seeds, crushed

1 tsp turmeric

½ tsp chili powder

400ml half-fat coconut milk

1 tbsp tamarind paste

1 tbsppeanut butter

coriander or breads or rice, to serve

Directions:

Heat 1 tbsp oil in a pan. Cook the aubergine in batches until golden and soft. Add another tbsp of oil if you need to. Scoop out once they are done.

Add the onion to the same pan and cook until soft and golden. Add the garlic and ginger and cook for a minute. Add the spices and cook for 2 minutes.

Tip in the coconut milk, tamarind and peanut butter. Simmer gently until the peanut butter dissolves. Add the aubergine back and simmer for 15 minutes. Stir through some coriander and serve with bread or rice.

Falafel mezze bowl

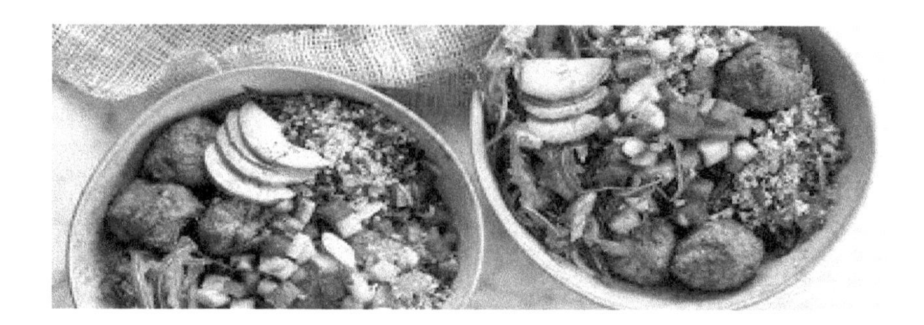

Preparation Time: 5 minutes

Cooking Time: 20 minutes

Servings: 2

Ingredients

olive oil

½ lemon, juiced

50g young spinach

4 tbsp hummus

2 roasted red peppers from a jar, sliced

1 tbsp pumpkin seeds, toasted

warm pitas, to serve

chili sauce to serve

200g falafel

Directions:

Heat the falafels in the oven, following packet instructions. Whisk 1 tbsp oil with 2 tbsp of lemon juice and season.

Dress the spinach and divide between 2 large bowls. Add the falafel, hummus and peppers in separate piles.

Scatter over the pumpkin seeds and serve with pitas and chili sauce.

Patties

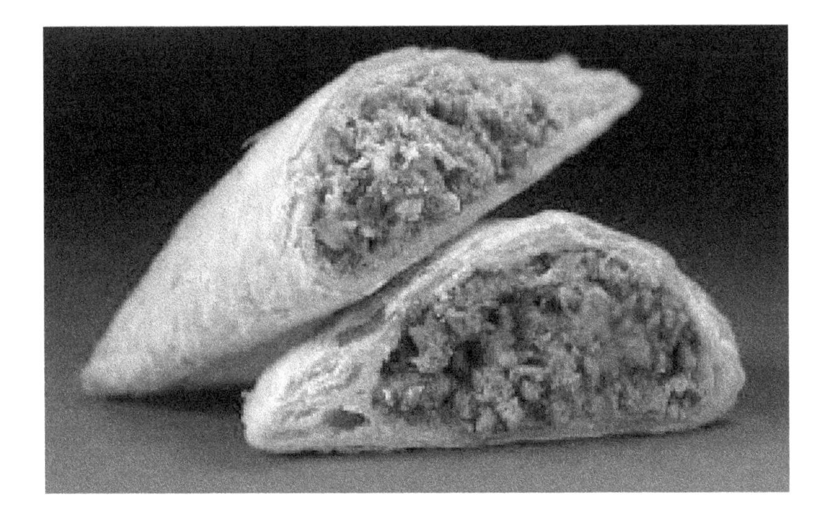

Preparation Time: 5 minutes

Cooking Time: 30 minutes

Servings: 2

Ingredients:

olive oil

1 garlic clove, crushed

2 carrots, diced small

2 celery sticks, diced small

1 large leek, chopped

900ml vegetable stock

1 tbsp tomato purée

3 tbsp pearl barley

1 x 400g tin borlotti beans

about 150g leafy greens, any woody stalks removed and shredded

crusty bread, to serve

Directions:

Heat 2 tbsp oil in a large pan then add the garlic, carrots, celery and leeks and cook until softened. Add the stock, tomato purée and barley. Bring to a simmer then cook for 15-20 minutes until barley is just tender. Add the beans and greens and simmer for 5 more minutes. Serve with crusty bread.

Cabbage with Coconut & Turnip

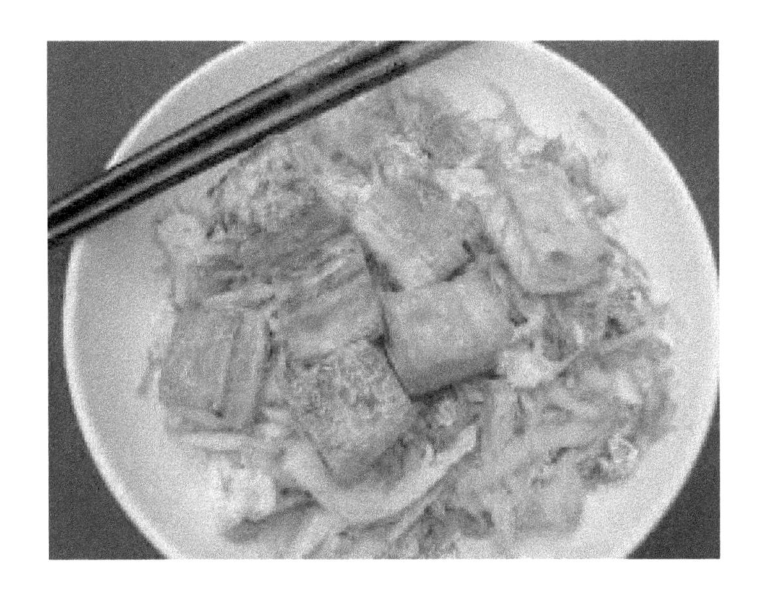

Preparation Time: 10 minutes

Cooking Time: 40 minutes

Servings: 2

Ingredients:

1 lb. unpeeled and halved turnips

2 tbsps. coconut oil

1 pinch Asafoetida

1 tsp. black mustard seeds

1 tsp. cumin seeds

2 dried red chilies

1 fresh seedless and thinly sliced red or green chili

1 finely shredded cabbage head

1/2 seville orange juice

2 tbsps. desiccated or shaved fresh coconut

Directions:

In a large pot, pour in water with salt then boil it.

Add the potatoes then stir.

Cook for about 10 minutes.

Drain the water then add them to a bowl.

Crush the potatoes with a fork gently.

In a skillet, heat the oil then add spices, the chilies, and Asafoetida.

Sauté for about 2 mins then toss in salt, fresh chili, and the cabbage.

Stir as you cook it for about 4 minutes.

Stir in the drained potatoes then cook for 3 minutes.

Add in the Seville orange juice, coriander, and coconut.

Properly mix them.

Serve warm with coconut yogurt.

Cauliflower Curry Soup

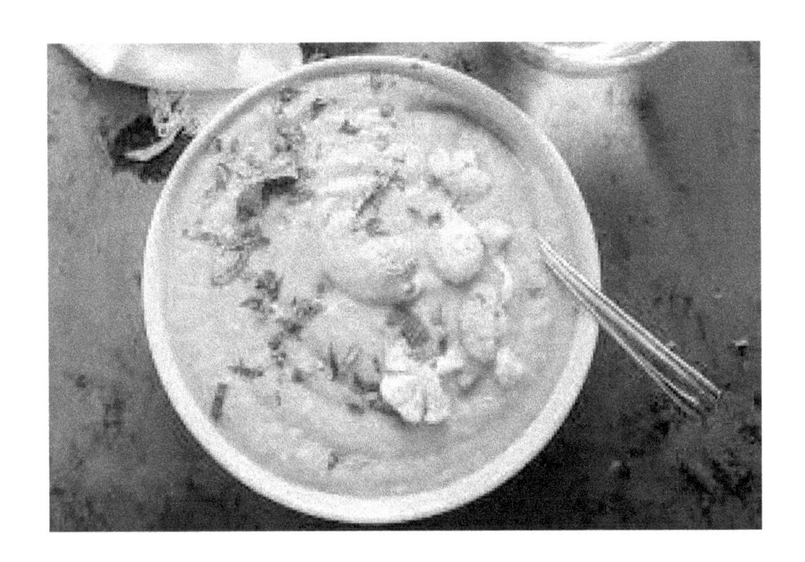

Preparation Time: 10 minutes

Cooking Time: 45 minutes

Servings: 4

Ingredients:

1 chopped large head of cauliflower

4 tbsps. divided coconut oil

1 diced medium yellow onion

3 tbsps. Thai red curry paste

1/2 tsp. Seville orange zcst

1/2 cup unoaked white wine

1-1/2 cups vegetable stock

14 oz. light coconut milk

3 tsps. rice vinegar

Iodine free Celtic sea salt

Freshly ground black pepper

1 tbsp. chopped fresh basil

Nuts

Directions:

Adjust the temperature of your oven to 400°F.

In a bowl, mix the cauliflower with coconut oil.

Pour it on a large baking sheet as you spread it.

Bake for 30 minutes.

In a Dutch oven, melt 1 tbsp. coconut oil.

Add onion with a dash of salt to sauté for 3 minutes.

Add in the curry paste and seville orange zest then stir.

Properly mix them then add wine.

Cook until it is completely absorbed

Add the vegetable stock, coconut milk, and the roasted cauliflower.

Cook for 10 minutes on low heat to simmer.

Pour the soup using a handheld blender after cooling it for about 5 minutes.

Add salt and pepper to season.

Garnish the meal with the nuts and basil.

Serve warm.

Zucchini Turnip Soup

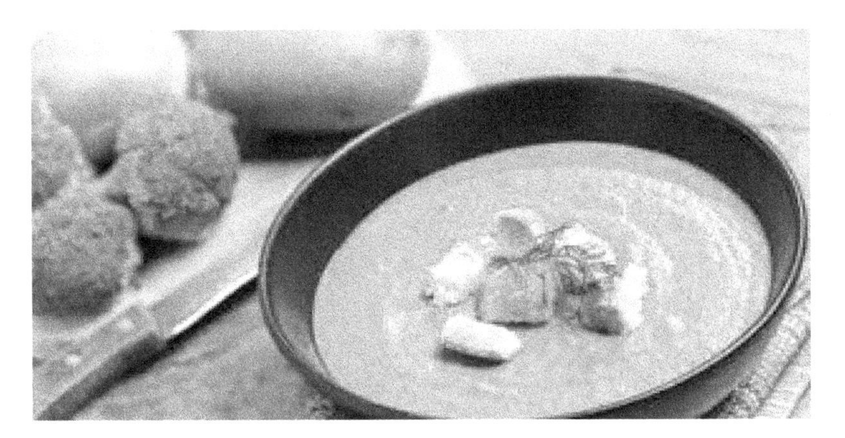

Preparation Time: 10 minutes

Cooking Time: 30 minutes

Servings: 4

Ingredients:

1 tbsp. coconut oil

2 cups chopped yellow onion

2 minced cloves chive

1 tbsp. minced fresh ginger

2 tbsps. red curry paste

4 cups low-sodium vegetable broth

3 cups peeled and diced zucchinis

3 cups peeled and diced turnips

Iodine free Celtic sea salt

Freshly ground black pepper

1/4 tsp. cayenne pepper

Directions:

Sauté the onion, ginger, and chive in a greased pan for about 6 minutes.

Add in the curry paste then stir and broth.

Mix properly then add the turnips, salt, and zucchinis

Boil the soup on high heat.

Cover the pot.

Cook for about 20 minutes.

Blend this soup in a blender in batches until it becomes smooth.

Add salt and pepper to season.

Serve warm.

Hot Dogs

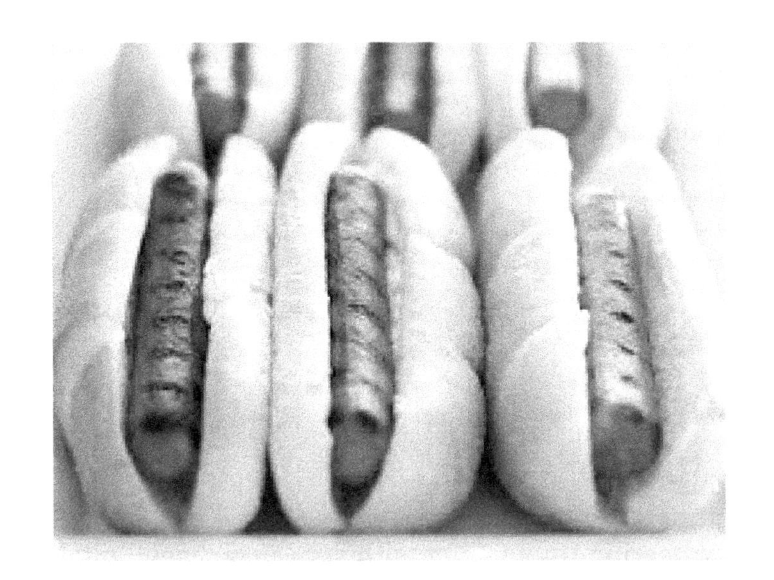

Preparation Time: 5 minutes

Cooking Time: 20 minutes

Servings: 2

Ingredients:

Grapeseed oil

Crushed red pepper, .5 tsp. – optional

Fennel, .5 tsp.

Dill, .5 tsp.

Ginger, .5 tsp.

Coriander, 1 tsp.

Diced shallots, .25 c

Diced onion, .33 c

Onion powder, 1 tbsp

Diced green bell pepper, .33 c

Smoked sea salt, 2 tsp.

Aquafaba, .5 c

Spelt Flour, 1 c

Garbanzo beans, 1 c

Directions:

Begin by heating up a skillet with some grapeseed oil and add in the vegetables and garbanzo beans. Sauté everything together for about five minutes until they are soft.

Add the vegetables into a food processor along with all of the other ingredients. Mix them all together until they are well blended. This is your hot dog mixture.

You can either use your hands or a hot dog mold for the next step. Take the mixture and mash it into a hot dog mold, or you can roll it into a hot dog shape using your hands. Wrap the hot dogs in some parchment paper.

Place a steamer basket inside a pot. Pour some water into the pot and boil the water. Lay the hot dogs on the steamer and let them steam for around 30 to 40 minutes. After they are done steaming, take the parchment paper off of them, or take them out of the mold.

To brown up the hot dogs, add some grapeseed oil to a skillet and brown for five to ten minutes. Enjoy your hot dogs on some Dr. Sebi approved hot dog buns with some alkaline ketchup.

Spring Rolls

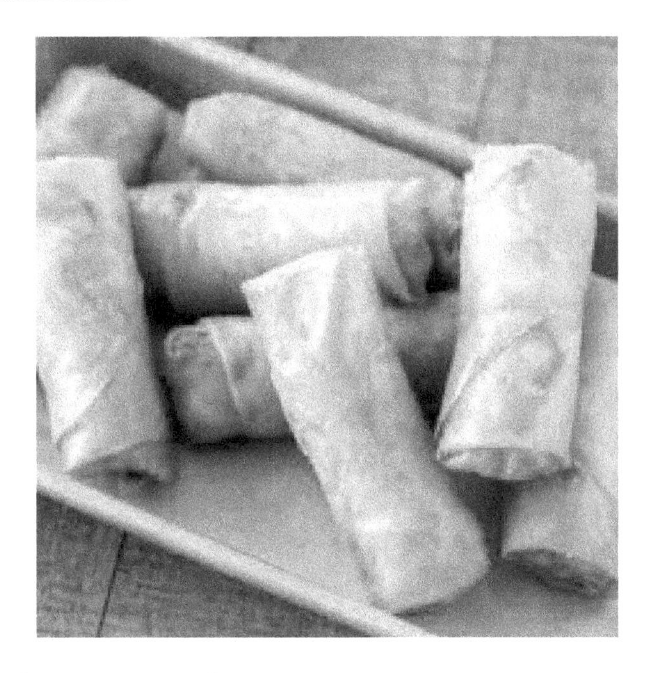

Preparation Time: 5 minutes

Cooking Time: 20 minutes

Servings: 2

Ingredients:

Kale Filling:

Grapeseed oil, 2 tsp.

Thinly sliced red bell pepper, .5

Onion powder, 1 tsp.

Sliced onion, .5 c

Kale, 3 c

Sea salt, 1 tsp.

Avocado Filling:

Sea salt, .5 tsp.

Diced green bell peppers, 2 tbsp

Onion powder, 1 tsp.

Diced red bell onion, 2 tbsp

Lime juice, 1 tsp.

Avocado

Spring Rolls:

Springwater, .5 c

Grapeseed oil, .33 c

Onion powder, 1 tsp.

Spelt Flour, 2 c

Sea salt, 1 tsp.

Directions:

Let's start by making the spring rolls. Add the seasonings and the flour to your food processor and mix everything together for about ten seconds. Slowly add in the grapeseed oil as it is mixing.

Slowly add in the water as it is mixing until a dough ball forms. Sprinkle your work surface with some flour and lay out the dough. Knead the dough until it comes together and then separate it out into five parts, as equal as you can.

Roll each of the sections out into a thin circle. Using a food scraper, cut out a six-inch square. Roll the cut off dough into a ball and continue to do this. Continue to make these squares until you have used up all of the dough. As you do this, place parchment paper between the dough so it doesn't stick.

Once the dough has been prepared, move onto getting the filling mixed together. For the kale filling, heat up a skillet and sauté everything together for about five to seven minutes, or until the veggies become tender.

For the avocado filling, slice the avocado in half, remove the pit, and then scoop out the filling. Add in all of the other ingredients and then mash everything together.

To assemble, brush the edges and corners of the dough with aquafaba before you roll it up so that it sticks together.

Add two to three tablespoons of a filling into the center of the dough. Pull the bottom corner up and over the filling and then fold in the right and left sides into the middle, and then roll up towards the top corner. You want it tight enough so that the filling doesn't fall out.

In a lightly greased skillet, place the egg roll in the pan and cook for about a minute on both sides. Once the sides are done, fry on the very ends of the roll. Enjoy.

Hummus

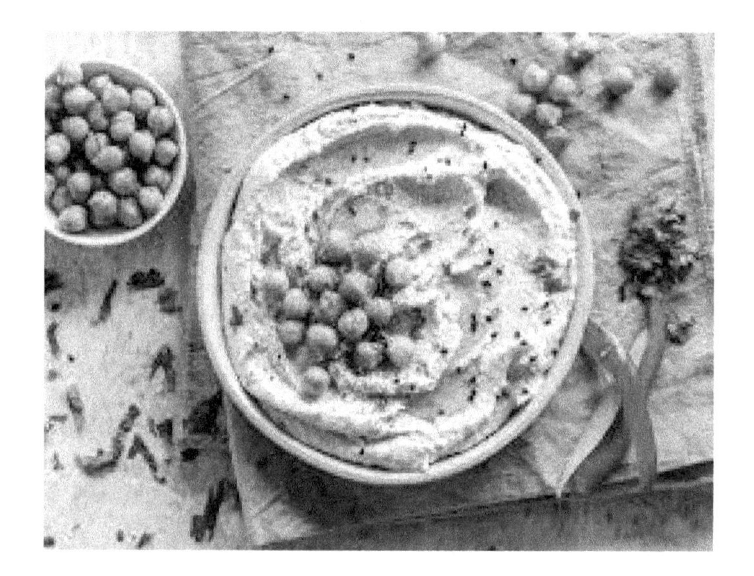

Preparation Time: 5 minutes

Cooking Time: 50 minutes

Servings: 2

Ingredients:

Sea salt, to taste

Onion powder, dash

Juice of one key lime

Tahini butter, .33 c

Olive oil, 2 tbsp

Cooked chickpeas, 1 c

Directions:

You will need to put the ingredients listed above into your blender. Turn the blender on and leave it on until creamy and smooth.

Crunchy Hummus

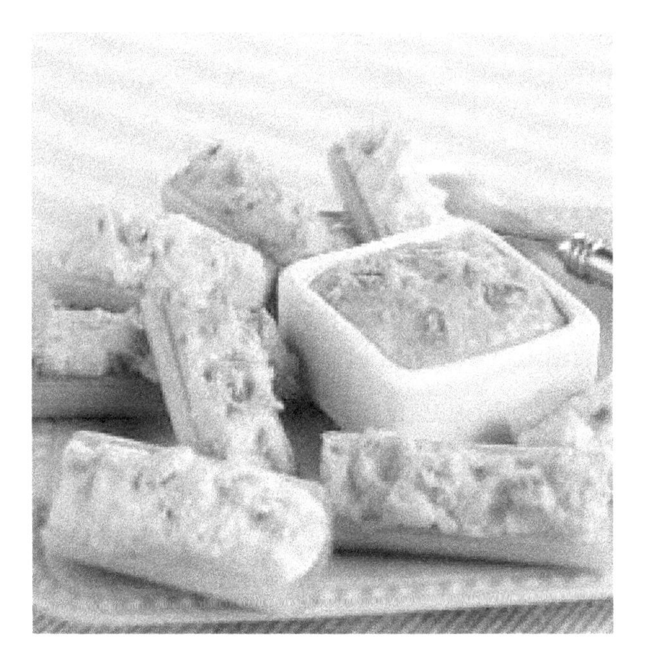

Preparation Time: 5 minutes

Cooking Time: 30 minutes

Servings: 2

Ingredients:

Red onion, .5

Fresh coriander, 2 tbsp

Cherry tomatoes, .25 c

Red bell pepper, .5

Dulse flakes, 1 tbsp

Juice of a lime

Sea salt

Olive oil, 3 tbsp

Tahini, 2 tbsp

Warm chickpeas, 1 c

Directions:

Start by warming your chickpeas. You can do this in a couple of different ways. You can place them on a baking sheet in an oven that has been heated to 250. Simply keep an eye on them, stirring them every five minutes or so until lightly warmed. You can also do this in a skillet. Stir the chickpeas every few minutes to make sure they don't burn until they are lightly warmed.

Then add your warmed chickpeas to a bowl along with the tahini, sea salt, and lime. With a fork, mash the chickpeas and ingredients together until it forms a paste. It doesn't have to be perfectly smooth.

Add in the chopped onion, cherry tomatoes, bell pepper, dulse flakes, and olive oil. Mix everything together until it is well combined. Enjoy this hummus on a couple of slices of organic spelt bread.

Vegetable Quinoa

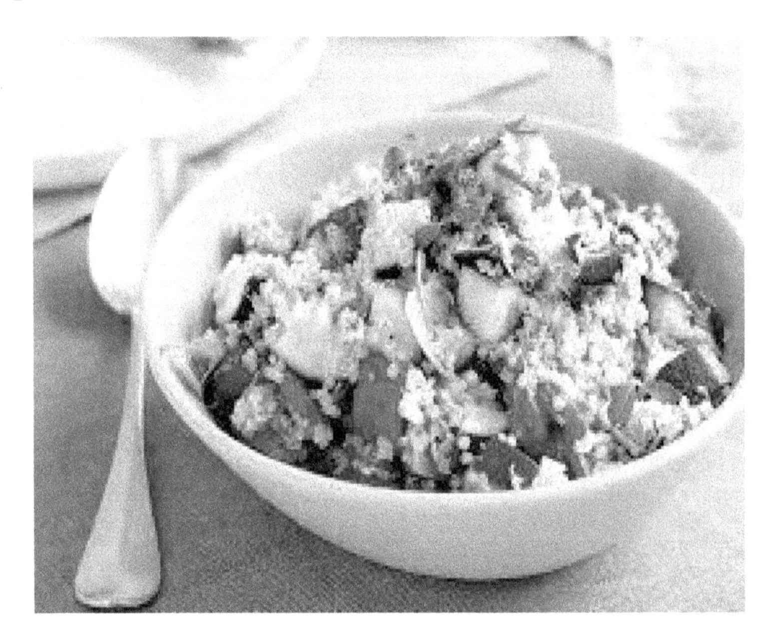

Preparation Time: 5 minutes

Cooking Time: 40 minutes

Servings: 2

Ingredients:

Cayenne, .5 tsp.

Grapeseed oil, 2 tbsp

Diced plum tomato

Oregano, 1 tsp.

Diced red onion, .5 c

Basil, 1 tsp.

Springwater, .5 c

Onion powder, 1 tsp.

Diced yellow bell pepper, .25 c

Sea salt, 2 tsp.

Diced green bell pepper, .25 c

Diced red bell pepper, .25

Chipped zucchini, 1 c

Cooked quinoa, 4 c

Directions:

Add your oil into a skillet. Add in the vegetables and the seasonings. Cook them for five to ten minutes.

Add quinoa and water. Stir well and cook for five minutes more. Enjoy.

Kamut Cereal

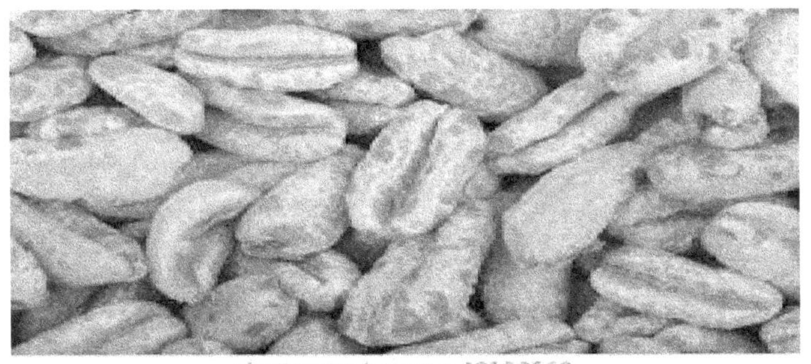

Preparation Time: 5 minutes

Cooking Time: 20 minutes

Servings: 2

Ingredients:

Sea salt

Oregano

Onion powder

Cayenne

Springwater, 2 c

Kamut, 1 c

Directions:

Pour the water into a pot and add in the sea salt. Leave alone until it begins to boil. Add a cup of the Kamut berries to a food processor and grind them up until they start to look like grits.

Add the Kamut into the boiling water. Constantly stir the Kamut as it is cooking. You can add more spring water when you need to in order to reach your desired consistency.

You can add in whatever seasoning you would like to and enjoy.

Snacks and desserts and smoothies

Spicy Green Smoothie

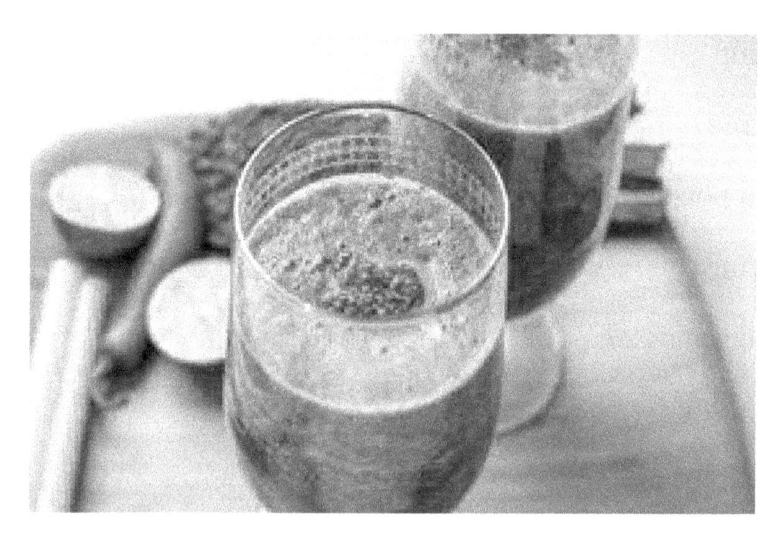

Preparation Time: 5 minutes

Cooking Time: 0 minutes

Servings: 2

Ingredients:

Sea moss gel, 1 tbsp

Lime juice, .25 c

Springwater, 2 c

Thumb of ginger

Cucumber, 1 c

Apple

Kale, 2 handfuls

Directions:

Add everything to your blender and mix for a couple of minutes, or until it is blended to your liking. Enjoy.

Crisp Green Smoothie

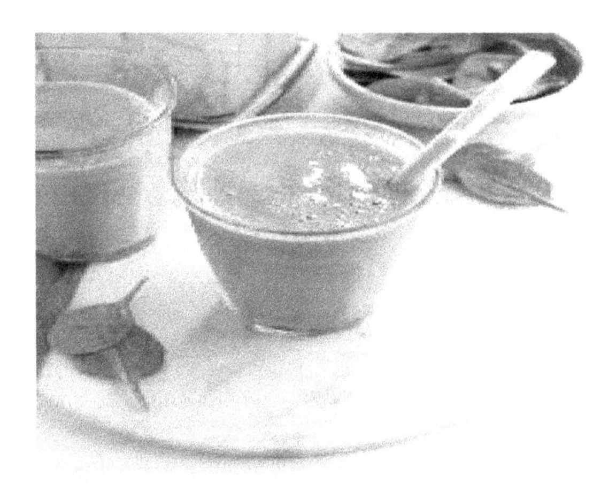

Preparation Time: 5 minutes

Cooking Time: 0 minutes

Servings: 2

Ingredients:

Sea moss gel, 1 tbsp

Lime juice, .25 c

Springwater, 2 c

Thumb of ginger

Dates, 6

Honeydew, .25

Cucumber, 1 c

Pear

Bunch of arugulas

Bunch of callaloo

Directions:

Add everything to your blender and mix for a couple of minutes, or until it reaches your desired consistency. Enjoy.

Fruity Green Smoothie

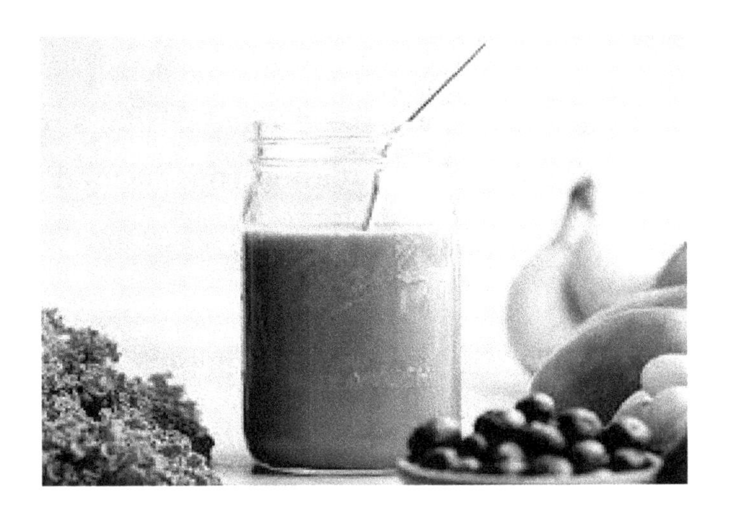

Preparation Time: 5 minutes

Cooking Time: 0 minutes

Servings: 2

Ingredients:

Burdock root powder, 1 tbsp

Lime juice, .25 c

Springwater, 2 c

Thumb of ginger

Dates, 6

Baby bananas, 3

Blueberries, .5 c

Handful of watercress

Bunch of dandelion greens

Directions:

Add all of the ingredients to a blender and mix for a couple of minutes, or until it reaches your desired consistency. Enjoy.

Triple Berry Smoothie

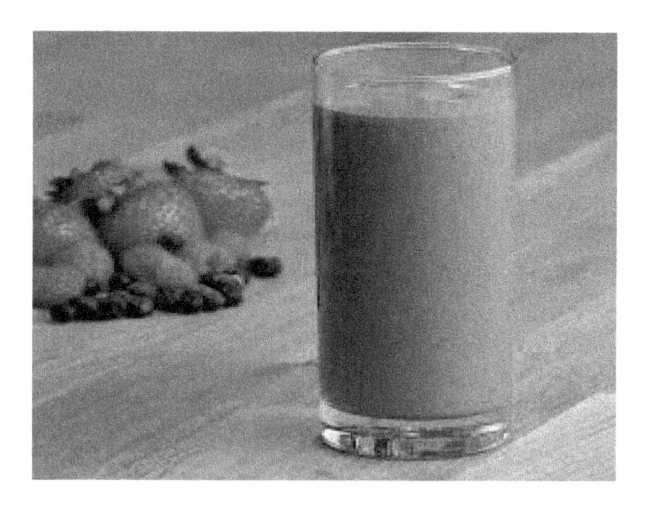

Preparation Time: 5 minutes

Cooking Time: 0 minutes

Servings: 2

Ingredients:

Agave

Burro banana

Water, 1 c

Blueberries, .5 c

Raspberries, .5 c

Strawberries, .5 c

Directions:

Begin by washing the fruit. Peel and dice the banana. Add the fruit to the blender. Begin blending and slowly add the water in until it reaches the consistency you like. Blend in some agave to taste.

Toxin Flush Smoothie

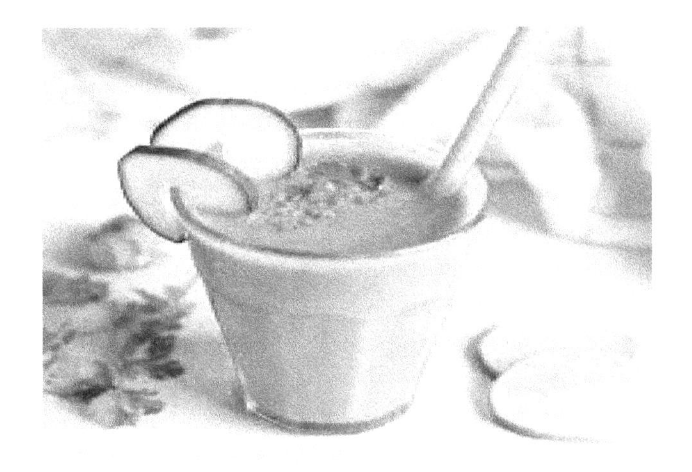

Preparation Time: 5 minutes

Cooking Time: 0 minutes

Servings: 2

Ingredients:

A key lime

A cucumber

Cubed, seeded watermelon, 1 c

Directions:

Wash and dice the cucumber. Add the watermelon and cucumber to the blender and mix until combined. You shouldn't need to add extra water since both the watermelon and cucumber are mainly water.

Slice the lime in half and squeeze the juice into your smoothie. Enjoy.

Detoxifying Smoothie

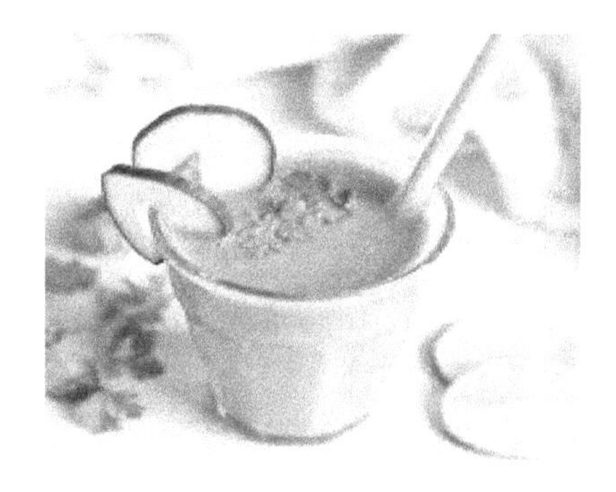

Preparation Time: 5 minutes

Cooking Time: 0 minutes

Servings: 2

Ingredients:

A key lime

A quarter of an avocado

Amaranth greens, 2 c

Cored apples, 2

Water, 2 c

Directions:

Begin by cleaning the apples and amaranth greens. If your blender is a high speed one, you should peel the apples first. Add the apples, greens, and avocado to a blender. Mix everything together in the blender and slowly add the water into the mixture until it reaches your desired consistency. Juice the lime into your smoothie and mix together.

Zucchini Pepper Chips

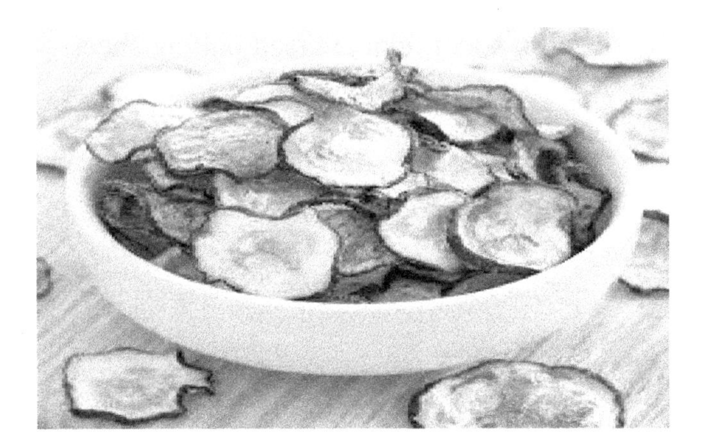

Preparation Time: 10 minutes

Cooking Time: 15 minutes

Servings: 4

Ingredients:

1-2/3 cups vegetable oil

1 tsp. onion powder

1/2 tsp. ground black pepper

3 tbsps. red pepper flakes, crushed

2 zucchinis, thinly sliced

Directions:

Mix the oil with all the spices in a bowl.

Then add the zucchini slices and mix well.

Transfer the mixture to a Ziplock bag then seal it.

Refrigerate the mixture for about 10 minutes.

Spread the zucchini slices on a greased baking sheet.

Bake for about 15 minutes.

Serve.

Apple Chips

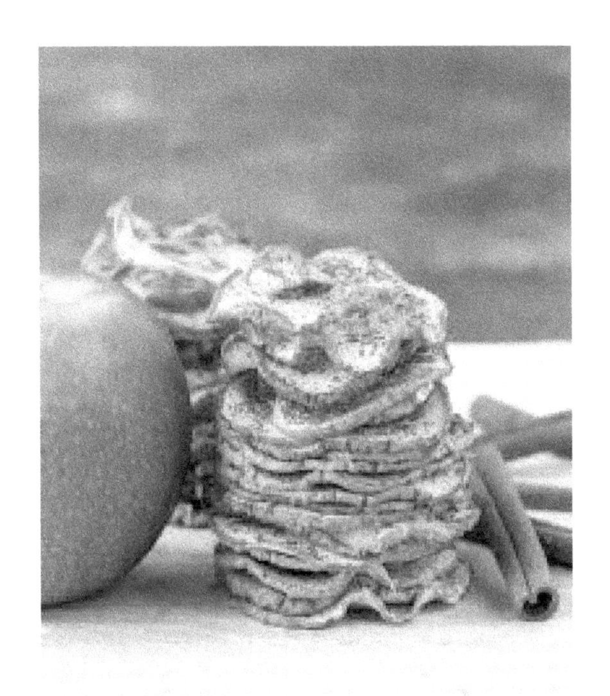

Preparation Time: 5 minutes

Cooking Time: 45 minutes

Servings: 4

Ingredients:

2 cored and thinly sliced Golden Delicious apples

1-1/2 tsps. date sugar

1/2 tsp. ground cinnamon

Directions:

Adjust the temperature of oven to 225°F.

Put the apple slices on a baking sheet.

Sprinkle the sugar on the apples.

Add cinnamon over apple slices.

Bake for about 45 minutes.

Serve.

Kale Crisps

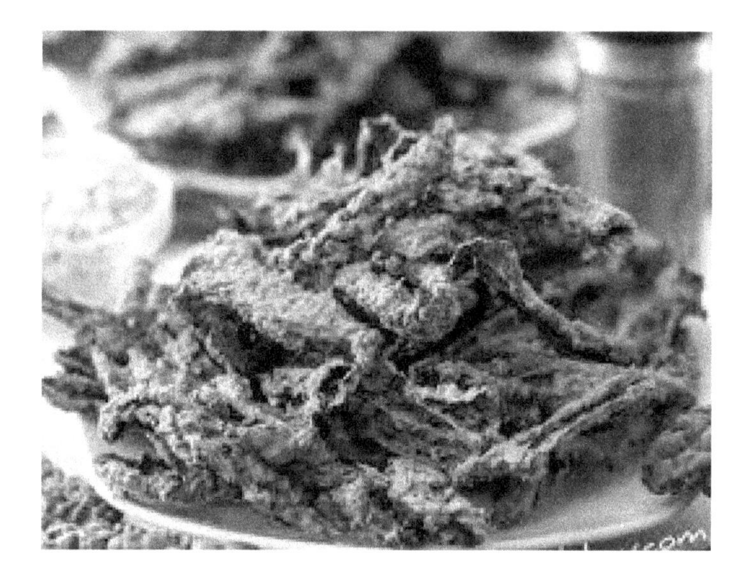

Preparation Time: 10 minutes

Cooking Time: 10 minutes

Servings: 4

Ingredients:

1 bunch kale with stems removed, leaves torn into even pieces

1 tbsp. olive oil

1 tsp. sea salt

Directions:

Adjust the temperature of your oven to 350°F.

Layer a baking sheet with parchment paper.

Spread the kale leaves on a paper towel to absorb the moisture.

Add salt and olive oil to the leaves.

Spread them on the baking sheet then bake for about 10 minutes.

Serve.

Turnip Chips

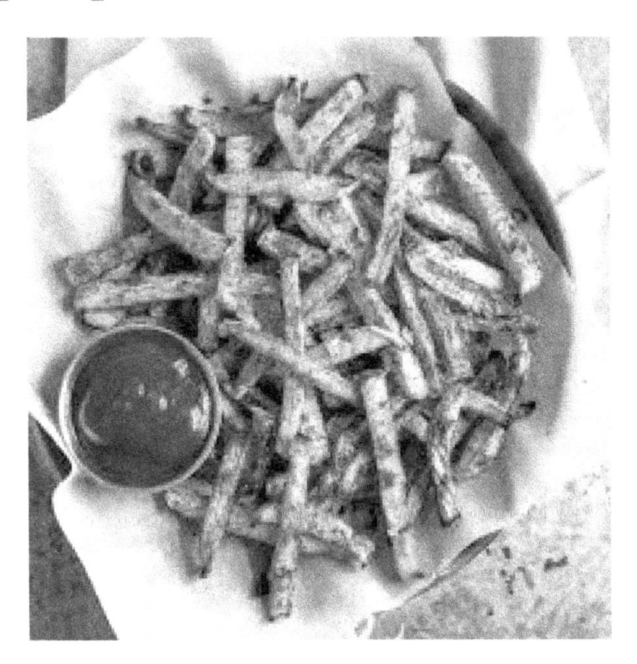

Preparation Time: 5 minutes

Cooking Time: 5 minutes

Servings: 4

Ingredients:

1 thinly sliced turnip

2 tsps. olive oil

Coarse sea salt

Directions:

Toss the turnip with oil and salt.

Spread the slices in a baking dish in a single layer.

Cook in a microwave for about 5 minutes until golden brown.

Serve.

Tortillas

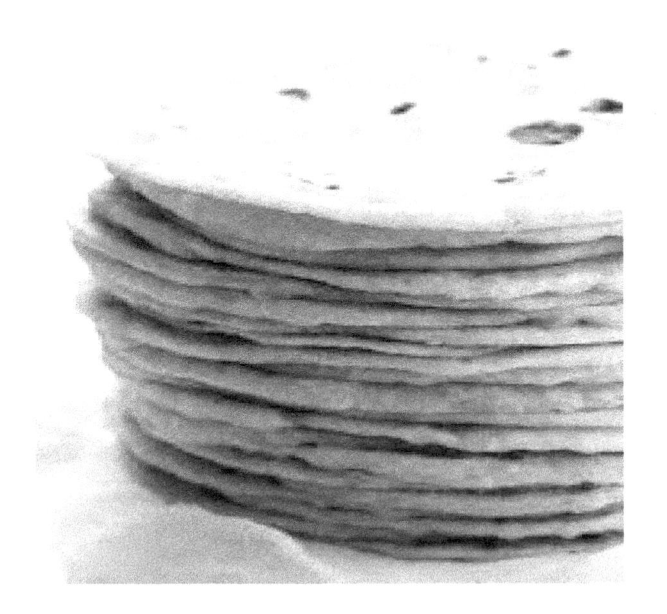

Preparation Time: 6 minutes

Cooking Time: 20 minutes

Servings: 8

Ingredients

2 cups Spelt Flour

1 tsp. Pure Sea Salt

1/2 cup Spring Water

Directions:

Mix the spelt flour with Pure Sea Salt in a food processor for about 15 seconds.

Continue blending as you slowly add the Grape Seed Oil until well incorporated.

Add the spring water slowly while blending until a dough is formed.

Prepare a work surface then cover it with a piece of parchment paper.

Sprinkle the paper with flour.

Knead the dough for about 2 minutes until it achieves the right consistency.

Divide the dough into 8 equal balls.

Roll out each ball into a very thin circle.

Preheat a non-stick pan, cook one tortilla at a time on moderate heat for about 60 seconds on every side.

Serve and enjoy.

Detox Berry Smoothie

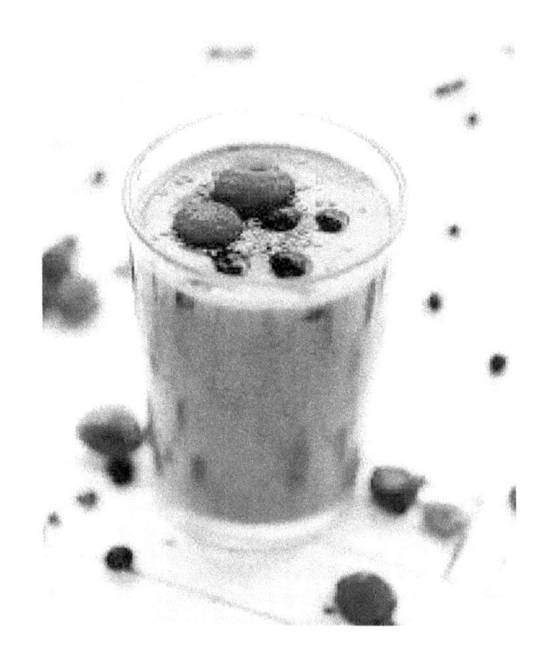

Preparation Time: 5 minutes

Cooking Time: 0 minutes

Servings: 2

Ingredients:

A quarter of an avocado

Water

Hemp seeds, 1 tbsp

Fresh lettuce, 2 c

Mixture of your favorite berries, 1 c

Seville orange

Burro banana

Directions:

Wash your berries. Peel the orange and banana. Segment the orange out and slice the banana. Add the berries, orange, banana, lettuce, and avocado to the blender. Start mixing them all together, and slowly add in the water until it reaches the consistency you like. Mix in the hemp seeds and enjoy.

Blissful Smoothie

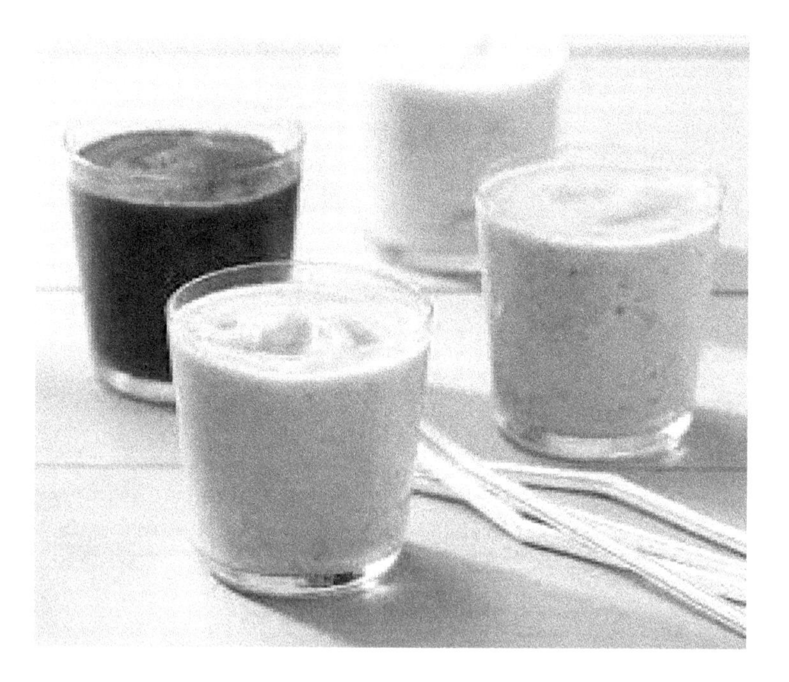

Preparation Time: 5 minutes

Cooking Time: 0 minutes

Servings: 2

Ingredients:

Water, 1 c

Cooked quinoa, .25 c

Blueberries, 1 oz

A quarter of an avocado

Chopped pear

Directions:

You first need to start by cooking your quinoa and allowing it to cool completely. This is a good recipe to do the morning after you have had quinoa for dinner.

Then wash your fruit and chop up the pear. Add the quinoa, blueberries, avocado, and pear to your blender. Being mixing everything together and slowly add in the water until it reaches your desired consistency. Enjoy.

Apple Blueberry Smoothie

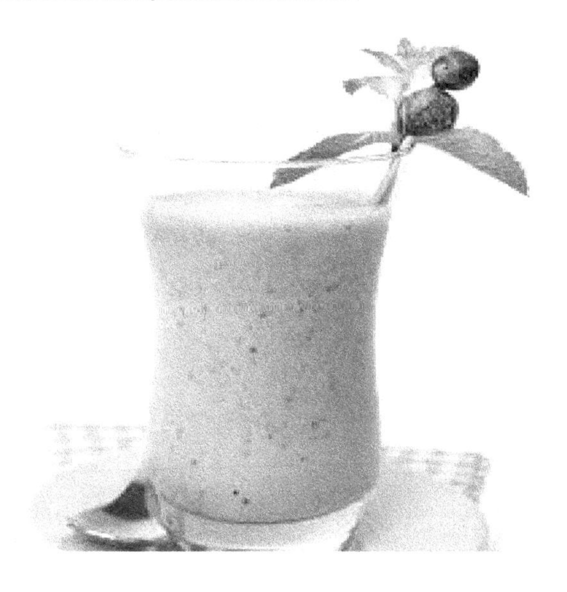

Preparation Time: 15 minutes

Cooking Time: 0 minutes

Servings: 2

Ingredients:

Bromide plus powder, .5 tbsp

A date

Sesame seeds, 1 tbsp

Soft-jelly coconut water, 2 c

Hemp seeds, 1 tbsp

Callaloo, .5 c

A half of an apple

Blueberries, .5 c

Directions:

Begin by washing and dicing your apple. You can also peel the apple if your blender doesn't mix things up perfectly. Wash the blueberries, and then add the fruit to your blender and along with all of the other ingredients. Mix everything together and enjoy.'

Green Veggie Berry Smoothie

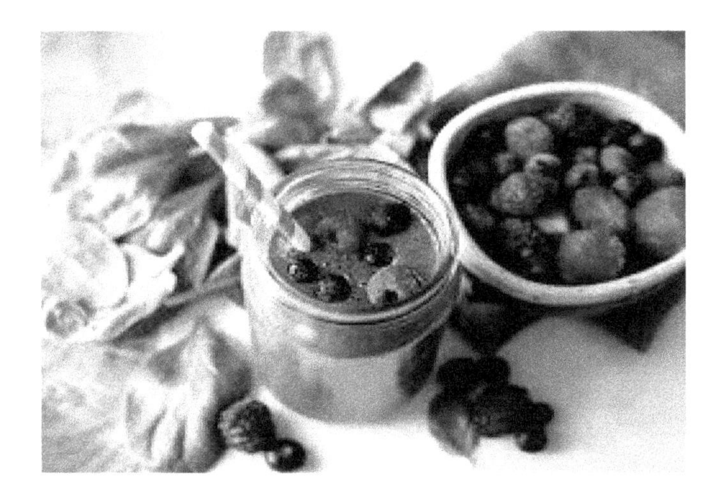

Preparation Time: 5 minutes

Cooking Time: 0 minutes

Servings: 2

Ingredients:

Springwater, 1 c

Handful of your favorite approved berries

Burro banana

Favorite approved greens, 2 c

Directions:

Begin by washing your berries and greens. Peel and slice your banana and then add all of the fruits and veggies into your blender. Begin to blend everything together and slowly add in the water until the smoothie reaches the consistency that you like. Enjoy.

Banana "Ice Cream" Smoothie

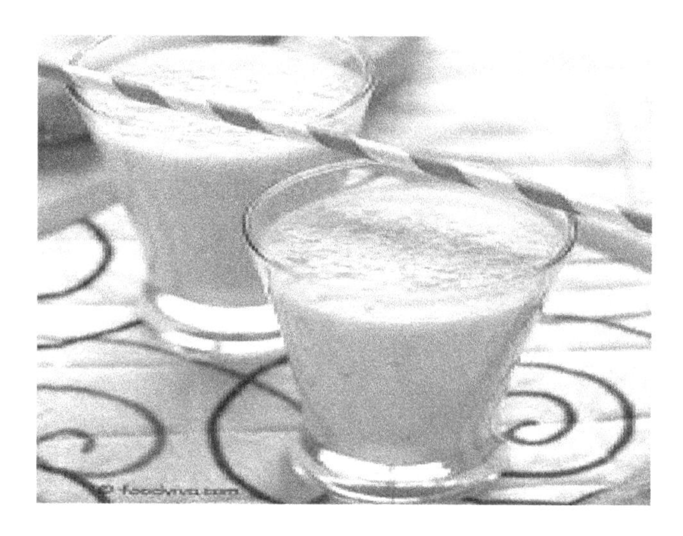

Preparation Time: 5 minutes

Cooking Time: 0 minutes

Servings: 2

Ingredients:

Ginger, .5 tsp.

Springwater, 1 c

Approved nut butter, 1 tbsp

A handful of raisins

Frozen, sliced burro bananas, 2

Directions:

Begin by placing the raisins into a bowl of water and allow them to soak for at least two hours. This will help the texture of a smoothie so that it doesn't become grainy.

Once the raisins have soaked long enough, add them along with the bananas, nut butter, and ginger to your blender. Begin blending everything together and slowly add in the spring water until it reaches your desired consistency. Enjoy.

Prickly Pear Smoothie

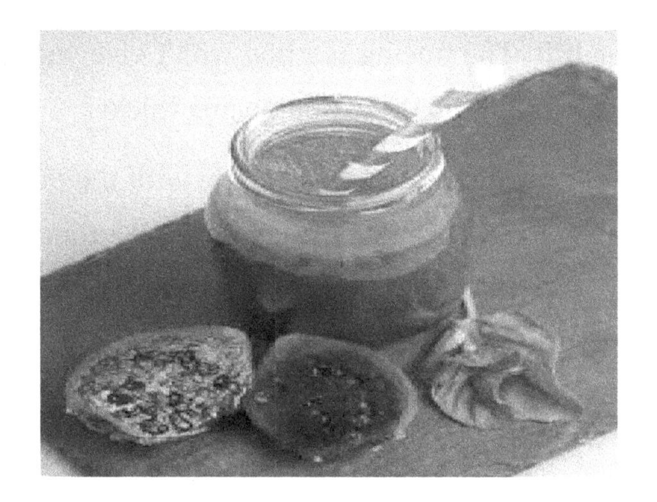

Preparation Time: 15 minutes

Cooking Time: 0 minutes

Servings: 2

Ingredients:

Ginger, .5 tsp.

Springwater, .5 c

Burro bananas, 2

Prickly pear juice, 1 c*

Directions:

First off, we will make the prickly pear juice.

You will take two prickly pears, make sure they are cleaned, and add them to your blender along with a cup of water. Mix everything together and then strain the juice through some cheesecloth. If you have a juicer, you can also run the prickly pears through it. The juicing method won't give you as much liquid, so your smoothie will end up being thicker.

Next, slice your bananas and them along with the prickly pear juice and ginger to your blender. Begin mixing them together and slowly add in the spring water until it reaches your desired consistency. Enjoy.

"Pretty in Pink" Smoothie

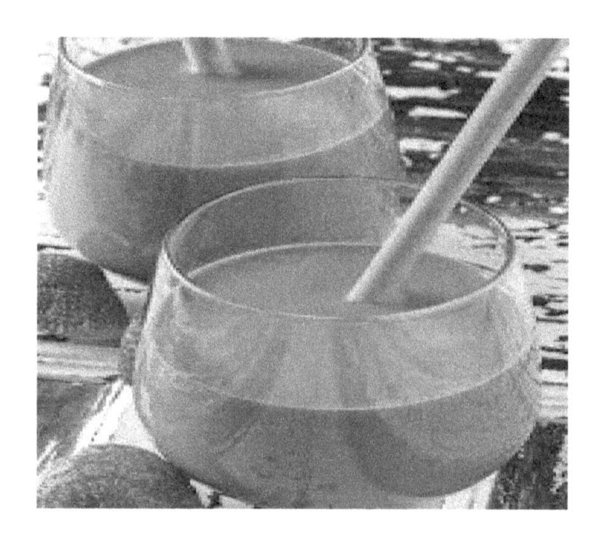

Preparation Time: 15 minutes

Cooking Time: 0 minutes

Servings: 2

Ingredients:

Burro banana

Small apple

A handful of your favorite berries, frozen

Directions:

First, you will want to make sure you wash your fruit before you place them in the freezer to freeze. Then peel and chop your apple and slice the banana. Add all of the fruit to your blender and mix everything together. If the smoothie is too thick for you, you can blend in some spring water to thin it out some. Enjoy.

Chapter 11: 7-Day Meal Plan

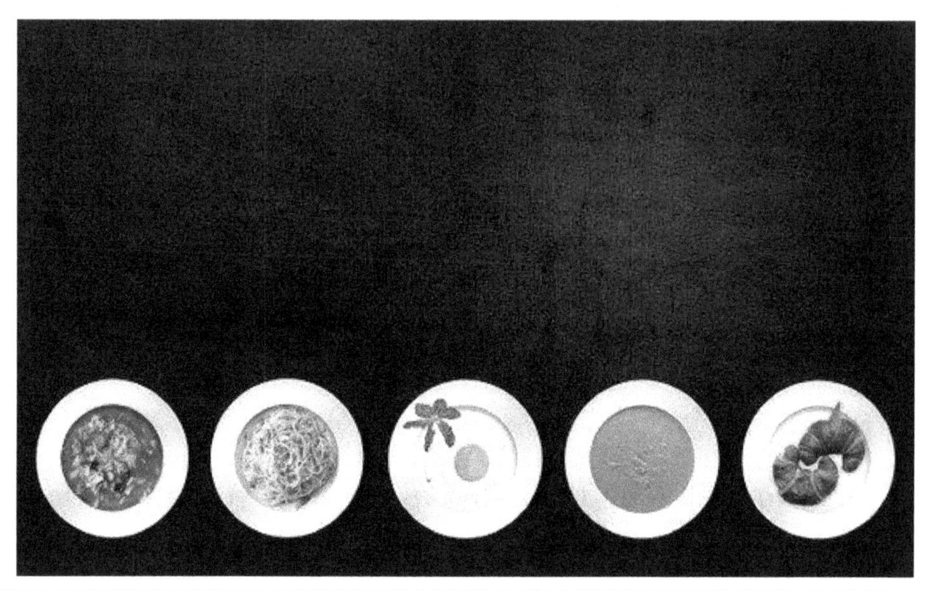

DAYS	BREAKFAST	LUNCH/DINNER	DESSERTS/SNACKS
1	Quinoa Porridge	Grilled Vegetable Stack	Spicy Green Smoothie
2	Zucchini Bread Pancakes	Bok Choy Soup	Crisp Green Smoothie
3	Hydrating Smoothie	Mushroom Cheese Steak	Fruity Green Smoothie
4	Juicy Portobello	Squash Falafels	Apple Chips

	Burgers		
5	Classic Homemade Hummus	Home Fries	Kale Crisps
6	Veggie Fajitas Tacos	Chicken Tenders	Blissful Smoothie
7	Amaranth Porridge	Veggies with Mushrooms	Apple Blueberry Smoothie

Chapter 12: Keys to Making Dr. Sebi's Diet a Success

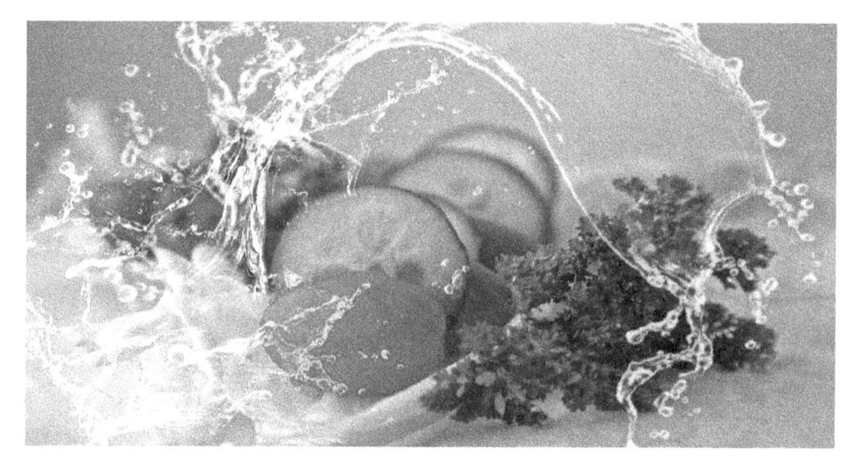

Dr. Sebi discovered many things during his lifetime. He also taught a lot of people many things. During his life, he did many interviews and performed at a lot of speaking engagements where he shared his secrets. Here, we will discuss his top ten diet secrets.

We have to go back to the mother

Dr. Sebi wrote a paper many years ago called Back to the Mother. In this, he talks about how the land provides for us in a specific manner. He speaks specifically about Africans and how they originally only had the land to live off of. That land provided the foods that they survived with, and that didn't include things like cows, potatoes, beans, yams, lambs, or rice. The lamb came from Arabia and the cow came from Europe.

The foods that they ate were electric, and that is what their body needs and that is what kept them healthy. Today, people have strayed from those ways because now they have access to foods from all over the world. Dr. Sebi explained this by saying that "you don't feed gorillas polar bear food." The problems we have are due to the fact that we have been given the wrong types of foods. This is the main point of his diet. He wants us to go back to the foods that our bodies want us to eat so that it is able to work properly and to its full capacity.

If you take a look at how other animals eat, you will start to notice something very different. Polar bears feed on seals. Hummingbirds feed on the nectar in flowers. Giraffes eat leaves. Among animals, you have herbivores and carnivores. But when it comes to humans, we don't eat the way our people ate centuries ago when food wasn't as prevalent. That means we aren't giving our bodies what it needs because we can't decide if we need meats or if we need herbs.

Fasting is key to healing your body from disease

When people hear the word fasting, they instinctively get defensive. When people think fasting, they think starvation, but that isn't what happens when you fast the Dr. Sebi way. Dr. Sebi fasted for 90 days and it helps to cure his diabetes and impotency. During those 90 days, he learned exactly what it was that people needed in order to heal. During this time, he began to drink his urine, lost his eyesight, but continued to do what he was supposed to be doing. Then, four days later his eyesight returned.

This is when he started to have everybody fast that was sick, which included his mother. This helped to cure her diabetes and cleared out her excess mucus in 57 days. Fasting does not mean that you give up food altogether. There are actually many different types of fast, and simply eating only the foods in his nutritional guide will put your body into a state of fasting. You can take things a step further by cutting out most foods except for dates when you are feeling rather weak and drinking bromide plus tea along with plain salads. Fasting is a wonderful thing, and you can experiment with fasting to see what works best for you.

Reading of the Ingredient labels

Avoiding other types of foods can be difficult most times. So, you can resort to reading the labels of the products to know the ingredients in them. It keeps you in the know-how of what you take into your body. The habit also assists in directing you in what to change from the foods you eat. It will also assist you once you have fully embraced Dr. Sebi's diet. Here, you will be in the know of whatever you consumed.

Drinking Plenty Water

According to the doctor, one should drink a gallon of spring water on the minimum daily. Avoid taking water containing softeners. Water from reverse osmosis systems should be avoided too. The work of the water is to help in nutrient absorption and organ and Joint cushioning. Remember that existing health organizations do recommend the intake of a gallon of water as well.

You should also make the drinking of the water to become a habit/culture.

Get Mentally and Emotionally Prepared

After you have already thought of your move to the alkaline dieting, look into the obstacles that will prevent you either psychologically or mentally in your transformation journey. With the knowledge in the distractions, chances of successfully getting inducted to the diet are high.

Don't Quit Snacks

Since you are not supposed to take packed snacks from the stores does not mean that you should stop consuming snacks. You just need to take snacks in the right way. You can try preparing some on your own. The snacks can be a mixture of raisins, walnuts, or other fruits that have been dried.

Review the Approved Foods

Look into the non-recommended foods in the diet. Avoid them in every possible way that you can. When you are prepared mentally for the recommended foods, you will easily get used to them.

Add Whole Foods to Your Daily Diet

Work very hard in completely substituting the processed meals with the whole foods. A lot of processed foods contain sugars that are enhanced. The sugars are considered very addictive as they can trigger cravings for the foods.

Cooking is Vital

When you have decided to follow Dr. Sebi's diet, you need to cook using the recipes recommended by him. The said guides provide people with the alkaline recipes making the technique easy to execute. The guides cover every topic in detail. As you begin meal preparations, you will learn how to use the approved ingredients for cooking the meals that you like.

The Body Works Properly Through Chemical Affinity

During the trial in the late '80s that Dr. Sebi had to face, he asked the judge if it wasn't true that science had proven the body was carbon-based, and that in order for a carbon-based being to function correctly it needs carbon-based foods. This is what science calls chemical affinity. The body is only able to accept things that it is made of, not something new or alien to it. The foods that are able to provide you with what your body needs are electric foods. The body likes these foods because it makes its chemical makeup.

There is Only One Disease, and That is Excess Mucus

While this is quite possibly the most controversial part of Dr. Sebi's teachings, he has said time and time again that the only disease is too much mucus. When it comes to diseases like diabetes, HIV/AIDS, lupus, and so on, they are created by the body creating too much mucus in a certain area. The body needs mucus, and it contains several mucous membranes that keep things lubricated. When we eat the wrong foods or do things that cause our bodies to become acidic, that mucus starts to grow. The illness that you develop will depend on where all of that mucus begins to grow.

For people with diabetes, the pancreas is where the mucous grows. For something like bronchitis, the mucus is in the lungs. During his trial in the '80s, he asked the judge if she had ever been to an AIDS ward, and she told him yes. Then he asked what the AIDS patients spit up, and she replied with "mucus." That is the basis for his diet is to cleanse the cells of all of this excess mucus to help heal the body from diseases.

Sick People Need Large Doses of Iron Phosphate

Dr. Sebi, when asked by potential patients where they should start, he always tells them to start taking iron, which is found in his Bio Ferra product. Iron phosphates are what help the cells to remain healthy once they have been freed of their excess mucus. Modern medicine tends to give people lots of ferrous oxides. Iron is the only magnetic mineral on the planet. Iron pulls all other minerals to it, so when you take iron, you are also taking all other minerals as well.

The Body is Not Designed to Become Sick

The body was not created for it to become sick. Birds don't get sick. Elephants don't get sick. They don't need a vet. Lions and giraffes don't need a vet, and neither do any of the natural animals. If this is true, then why do humans get sick so often? Why do we suffer from problems like hay fever and allergies? We have violated the laws of nature. We would all probably be happy and okay with this as long as we remain happy until the day we die. But the thing is, we don't stay happy until the day we die. Because of the violation, we have made it has stressed our mind and our body. If you stay in this violation, you will be stressed until the day you die.

Carbon, Hydrogen, and Oxygen are the Main Players in Maintaining Life

This may seem extremely obvious because we are taught this in elementary science classes. Everything that the Universe creates is made up of carbon, hydrogen, and oxygen. Those are the main players in making something organic, and these are often missing from things that are created in a lab. These substances do not have starch in them. All substances that are created by Universe, and that are organic, will not contain starch.

All of these foods that are naturally present on the Earth, that was made the Universe, are all alkaline foods. These are all-natural. Our blood and body prefer to be fed by these foods because it does not like starch. Starch is only present because it binds things together. Things only have to be bound together if they are not meant to naturally be together.

You Have to Cleanse and Then Rebuild the Body

Dr. Sebi's diet works in two parts. First, when you start following his diet you will be cleansing your cells, which he called inter-cellular cleansing. This is what removes toxins and impurities from your body, which will in turn help to heal you from any diseases you are suffering from. Once the cells in your body have been cleansed, it will move into the second part, which rebuilding the body. This means that the body is brought back to its optimal functioning, and most likely to a state that you have never known. The best way for your body to be able to rebuild itself is through the use of iron. If you make sure that your iron level is where it is supposed to be, then you cannot get sick.

Spinach is Not a True Iron-Rich Food Because it is Not Alkaline

As you know already, iron is a very important part of Dr. Sebi's diet. Most everybody will tell you that spinach is a great source of iron, but Dr. Sebi will tell you it is not. Spinach is acidic food. It falls below a 6 on the pH scale because it has a starch base. That means it is not natural. The Universe didn't naturally make this so it is not a good source of iron and will not help your body in any way. On the other hand, moringa has 25 times the amount of iron than spinach does and is not acidic. It also has 14 times the amount of calcium as milk.

Conclusion

Thank you for making it through to the end of Dr. Sebi's treatments and cure. Let's hope it was informative and able to provide you with all of the tools you need to achieve your goals, whatever they may be.

Many people claim that the way we live in a culture today is incredibly harmful to our wellbeing. They conclude that consuming highly acidic products affects the quality of cells and body fluids. Sadly, this evidence was not applied to clinically in several clinical studies, although there were a variety of individuals who attempted alkaline diets and recorded impressive health benefits.

Alkaline diets can give some of their health benefits: decreased vitality, weight control, lower dependency or no insulin reliance on patients with diabetes, no acid reflux, enhancement in their hair, nails, eyes, better moods for sleep, mental stability, candida symptoms relief and just to name a couple.

Many people claim that his diet improved their health by using his compounds, and the herbal approach to heal the body worked better than any medical approach ever did. You can find many of his thoughts about herbal therapy and nutritional compounds on YouTube that help promote and teach healthy living long after his death.

If you can switch from your normal diet that is full of fast foods, saturated fats, refined sugars, and grains to Dr. Sebi's diet could actually help you lose some weight—increasing your intake of whole grains, vegetables, and fruits while getting rid of pork and beef can decrease your risk of elevated cholesterol, high blood pressure, Type 2 diabetes, heart disease, and cancer. Most people eat way too much sodium, and this diet can drastically reduce lower this amount. This, in turn, can help you lower your blood pressure, and this reduces your risk of heart disease and stroke.

Dr. Sebi's diet encourages eating healthy fats like plant oils, seeds, and nuts along with whole grain that is rich in fiber. These foods have a lower risk of developing heart disease.

Any diet that limits processed foods can help you have a better quality of diet.

Good luck to everyone who has decided to embark on the journey of alkaline dieting! I hope that you carefully follow the instructions of this diet to get closer to your desires and healthy life!

CPSIA information can be obtained
at www.ICGtesting.com
Printed in the USA
BVHW081536181120
593626BV00006B/251